Neuro Spinal Surgery
Operative Techniques
Lateral Mass Fixation in Sub-axial Cervical Spine

Neuro Spinal Surgery Operative Techniques
Lateral Mass Fixation in Sub-axial Cervical Spine

JKBC Parthiban

MCh (Neurosurgery) FNS Japan (Fujita)
Senior Consultant Neurosurgeon
Spine Neurosurgery
Kovai Medical Center and Hospital
Coimbatore, Tamil Nadu, India

Editor-in-Chief
Journal of Spinal Surgery (JOSS)

Past President
Neuro Spinal Surgeons' Association, India (NSSA)
Founder Member NSSA
Teaching Faculty AO Spine

Foreword
PS Ramani

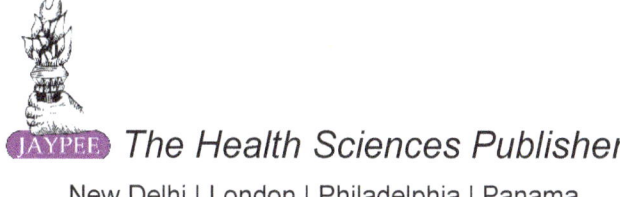

JAYPEE *The Health Sciences Publisher*

New Delhi | London | Philadelphia | Panama

Jaypee Brothers Medical Publishers (P) Ltd.

Headquarters
Jaypee Brothers Medical Publishers (P) Ltd.
4838/24, Ansari Road, Daryaganj
New Delhi 110 002, India
Phone: +91-11-43574357
Fax: +91-11-43574314
E-mail: jaypee@jaypeebrothers.com

Overseas Offices

J.P. Medical Ltd.
83, Victoria Street, London
SW1H 0HW (UK)
Phone: +44-20 3170 8910
Fax: +44(0) 20 3008 6180
E-mail: info@jpmedpub.com

Jaypee-Highlights Medical Publishers Inc.
City of Knowledge, Bld. 237, Clayton
Panama City, Panama
Phone: +1 507-301-0496
Fax: +1 507-301-0499
E-mail: cservice@jphmedical.com

Jaypee Medical Inc.
The Bourse
111, South Independence Mall East
Suite 835, Philadelphia, PA 19106, USA
Phone: +1 267-519-9789
E-mail: jpmed.us@gmail.com

Jaypee Brothers Medical Publishers (P) Ltd.
17/1-B, Babar Road, Block-B, Shaymali
Mohammadpur, Dhaka-1207
Bangladesh
Mobile: +08801912003485
E-mail: jaypeedhaka@gmail.com

Jaypee Brothers Medical Publishers (P) Ltd.
Bhotahity, Kathmandu, Nepal
Phone: +977-9741283608
E-mail: kathmandu@jaypeebrothers.com

Website: www.jaypeebrothers.com
Website: www.jaypeedigital.com

© 2016, Jaypee Brothers Medical Publishers

The views and opinions expressed in this book are solely those of the original contributor(s)/author(s) and do not necessarily represent those of editor(s) of the book.

All rights reserved. No part of this publication may be reproduced, stored or transmitted in any form or by any means, electronic, mechanical, photocopying, recording or otherwise, without the prior permission in writing of the publishers.

All brand names and product names used in this book are trade names, service marks, trademarks or registered trademarks of their respective owners. The publisher is not associated with any product or vendor mentioned in this book.

Medical knowledge and practice change constantly. This book is designed to provide accurate, authoritative information about the subject matter in question. However, readers are advised to check the most current information available on procedures included and check information from the manufacturer of each product to be administered, to verify the recommended dose, formula, method and duration of administration, adverse effects and contraindications. It is the responsibility of the practitioner to take all appropriate safety precautions. Neither the publisher nor the author(s)/editor(s) assume any liability for any injury and/or damage to persons or property arising from or related to use of material in this book.

This book is sold on the understanding that the publisher is not engaged in providing professional medical services. If such advice or services are required, the services of a competent medical professional should be sought.

Every effort has been made where necessary to contact holders of copyright to obtain permission to reproduce copyright material. If any have been inadvertently overlooked, the publisher will be pleased to make the necessary arrangements at the first opportunity.

Inquiries for bulk sales may be solicited at: jaypee@jaypeebrothers.com

Neuro Spinal Surgery Operative Techniques
Lateral Mass Fixation in Sub-axial Cervical Spine

First Edition: **2016**

ISBN: 978-93-5250-052-9

Dedicated to
My parents Dad—Dr JKB Chandra (Late) and
Mom—Jayalakshmi (Late)
for shaping me to become a doctor and
to my family: My dearest wife Harini and son Pranai

Foreword

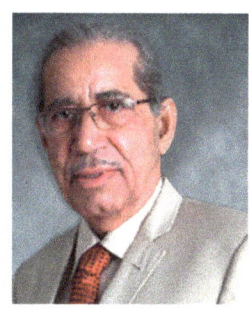

The understanding and development of spinal biomechanics and surgery started with lumbar spine. It took several decades before the interest was focused on the cervical spine and the surgical techniques on thoracic spine were last to be developed. The advent of minimally invasive spine surgery (MISS) and mesmerizing advance in technology the surgical techniques on spine were developed and are being practiced in leaps and bounds. Today cervical spine forms an important contribution to the day-to-day surgical procedures of any senior spinal surgeon all over the world. It was thus felt necessary by Dr JKBC Parthiban to bring out the book encompassing all the intricate surgical points that are needed to insert a successful lateral mass screw.

Younger spinal surgeons are doing a microdiscectomy in the lumbar spine. The experience gained will help a lot to achieve excellence in cervical lateral mass surgery. Being a new branch, the cumulative experience may not be rich but the developments have been so vast that it has attracted the attention of spinal surgeons very quickly and procedures like endoscopic cervical microdiscectomy, robot-assisted cervical discectomy, endo micro approach to the anterior and posterior cervical spine, etc. has become a reality.

Developments in cervical spinal stabilization have helped immensely to achieve progress in deformity reconstruction surgery which has now become an established discipline in cervical spinal surgery. Lateral mass stabilization with screws and rods is one such example. My colleagues and I feel immensely satisfied with the outcome as the contribution has been visionary.

With advance in medicine, the cervical spinal surgery has rapidly progressed and is today recognized as one of the most popular branches of spinal surgery after lumbar spine.

Fast pace and competitive spirit in day-to-day work unfortunately accelerates degeneration in the cervical spine and we see a lot of patients in the out-patient department with pain in the neck due to cervical spondylosis. The degeneration is so much advanced that decompression and stabilization appears to be in order. Posterior decompression and lateral mass stabilization is an excellent and safe technique to achieve this.

It is my ambition that this book should prove useful to guide all new spinal surgeons. I feel confident that it will be well received by the readers and particularly the younger generation of spinal surgeons all over the world. Continuous medical updates are mandatory to maintain the standards of practice. Similarly, in today's world, the experience of any spinal surgeon should never depend on a single teacher. The author Dr Parthiban is very meticulous and precise as well as thoughtful in making this book a useful guide. It will help them to provide better care to their patients. I feel very happy that Dr JKBC Parthiban has ventured to bring out this book in right time for the younger generation to learn and acquire this useful technique in cervical spinal stabilization.

Professor PS Ramani
MS CRCS (Lond) MSc Neuro (Eng) FICS FICA (USA) DSc FNAMS (Ind)
Senior Consultant Neuro and Spinal Surgeon
Lilavati Hospital and Research Center, Mumbai
Retired Professor and Head, Department of Neuro Spinal Surgery
University of Mumbai, Maharashtra, India
Founder and Honorary President
Neuro Spinal Surgeons' Association of India
Founder and Past President
Neuro Trauma Society of India
Past Chairman, World Federation of Neurosurgical Societies
Spine Committee
Founder Member, Asian Young Neuro Surgeons' Forum
Executive Committee Member, Asia-Pacific Non-Fusion Society
Past International President , Lumbar Fusion Society
Past President, Bombay Neurosciences Association
Member, WFNS Neuro Trauma Executive Committee
Founder and Editor-in-Chief, Journal of Spinal Surgery
Editor-in-Chief, Indian Edition of American Journal SPINE
Author of 44 books
Social Worker

Preface

Lateral mass fixation is not a new technique. However, ever since, I presented the first video of this technique in 1995 during the Neuro Trauma conference in Cochin, I see an overwhelming acceptance all over India. Many books and illustrations have been published on this subject.

There was a need for a simple illustrative book to show this technique done Step by Step for the young and practicing spine surgeons. Realizing this and understanding the need of younger generations during many cadaver dissection workshops, I decided to bring out an ideal book that would satisfy many surgeons.

While preparing this book, I kept one important point in my mind that I should deliver whatever I needed when I was a beginner in this subject. Though late this book has taken its shape at last and I am sure this may not be the last one from me. Many may come in future.

The take home message at the end is that the superolateral quadrant of the lateral mass of sub-axial cervical spine is the safest to place a screw and it is simple and safe.

Books are not written to be followed blindly. Surgeons are requested to go through it leisurely but at the same time cautiously and then practice with care and guidance. In case of doubt, no time should be wasted to communicate with me for clarification. My best wishes to all who are going to be benefitted by this small book.

Finally, we live to transfer our knowledge to others for the benefit of mankind.

JKBC Parthiban

Acknowledgments

Nothing is possible without my patients who had faith in me. This book is no exception. I am greatly indebted to all of them who extended their cooperation for this venture.

I thank the staff and management of Medical Trust Hospital, Cochin, Global Hospital, Chennai and Kovai Medical Center Hospital, Coimbatore, Tamil Nadu, for their support.

My special thanks to my nursing staff and theater technicians for their whole-hearted involvement.

The high quality pictures were taken by the team from Mr Anand's Video Vision, Coimbatore. Their commitment to the profession was great and I appreciate their cooperation.

Mr Samuel Williams, Gesco-Chennai is instrumental in arranging the instruments, implants and the bone models for the project. Many thanks to him.

I am grateful to Shri Jitendar P Vij (Group Chairman) and Mr Ankit Vij (Group President) of M/s Jaypee Brothers Medical Publishers (P) Ltd, New Delhi, India. My special thanks to Mr Tarun Duneja (Director–Publishing) and Mrs Samina Khan (Executive Assistant to Director–Publishing) for their kind cooperation in helping us to publish this edition in time. Finally, my sincere thanks to all the associates of the company with special mention to Mr KK Raman (Production Manager).

Mr Sabarish (Commissioning Editor), Jaypee Brothers Medical Publishers (P) Ltd., was in constant touch until the last moves were made to get the book completed.

My special thanks to Mrs Chetna (Associate Director–Content Strategy) for her immense help in shaping and bringing out the book in this present shape. I also thank all the other staff involved in designing and printing.

Contents

Section 1: BASICS

1. Surgical Anatomy of Lateral Mass   3
2. Landmarks   7
3. Neurovascular Structures in Relation to Lateral Mass   9
4. Standard Screw Trajectories   13

Section 2: SURGICAL TECHNIQUES

5. Positioning the Patient   19
6. Exposure   23
7. Drilling   32
8. Instrumentation   37
9. Case Reports   44
       Case 1   *44*
       Case 2   *47*
       Case 3   *48*
       Case 4   *52*
       Case 5   *56*
       Case 6   *59*

Index   *61*

Introduction

Lateral mass fixation with screws and rods in sub-axial cervical spine (C3–C6) is an elegant and effective technique performed through a posterior approach. It is easy to perform for inexperienced hands and easy to learn too. Practicing the technique in saw bone model and cadaver will help the young surgeons.

Roy Camille, a French orthopedic surgeon, popularized this technique. Magerl's modified the technique with changes in the screw trajectory using longer screws and gaining bicortical purchase of the lateral mass and claimed biomechanical superiority. Plates and monoaxial screws are now replaced with polyaxial screws and rods making the procedure very simple.

In this book, the technique of lateral mass fixation is described methodically for the readers to understand easily using simple language. The book is divided into two sections viz. Basics and Surgical Techniques and ends with illustrative cases. Readers are also encouraged to refer various textbooks and literature on this subject to enjoy this book.

Section 1

Basics

Chapter 1

Surgical Anatomy of Lateral Mass

An understanding of the anatomical relationships of the lateral masses of the cervical spine is very important to achieve proper screw placement. Since the surgeon visualizes only the posterior aspect of these masses, those structures that are immediately anterior to them are of prime concern when the screws are placed. The lateral mass (articular pillar) is the bulky lateral extension of the lamina and is connected to the vertebral body through the pedicles in an antero medial direction **(Figs 1.1A and B)**.

The transverse process, which harbors the foramen transversarium in its medial part, is connected to the vertebral body through a thin strut. It is also connected to the lateral mass through a relatively thicker bony portion **(Fig. 1.2)**. The lateral masses are called articular pillars **(Fig. 1.3A)**, since the superior and the inferior articular processes are formed from these masses**(Figs 1.3B and C)**. The superior facets are usually not seen from

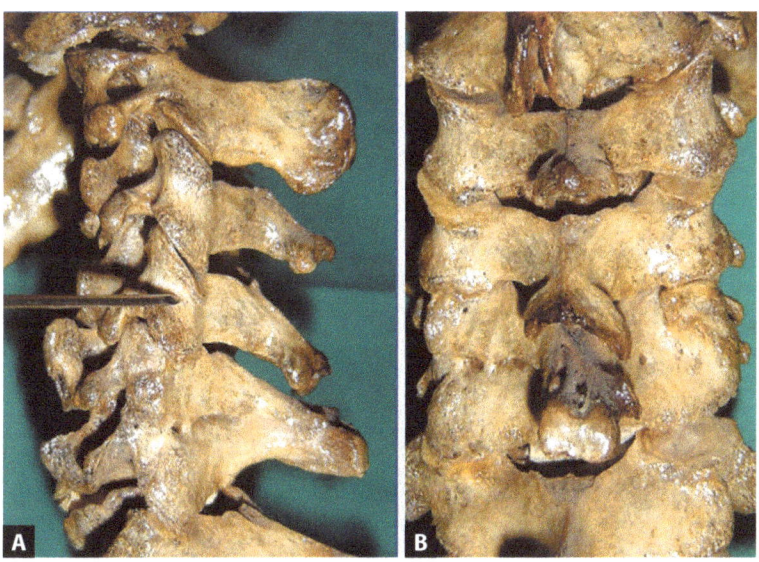

Figs 1.1A and B Lateral mass

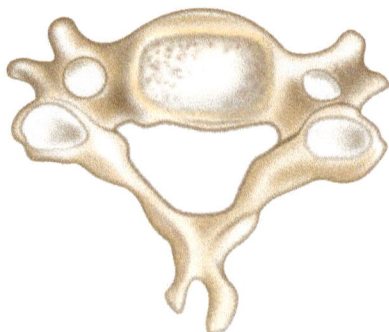

Fig. 1.2 Superior view of a typical subaxial cervical spine

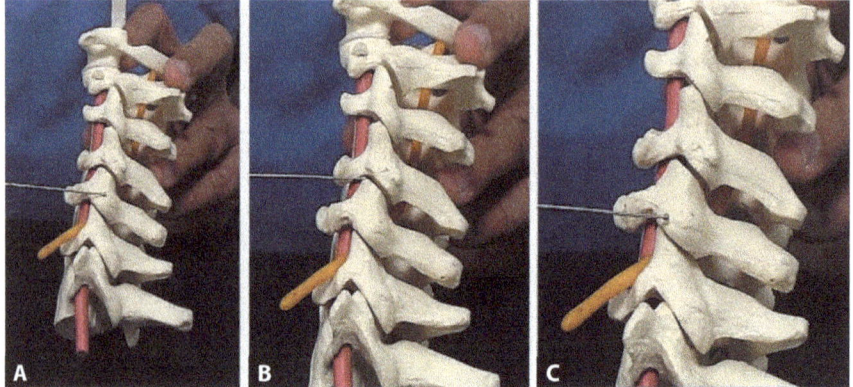

Figs 1.3A to C (A) Articular pillar; (B) Superior articular facet; (C) Inferior articular facet

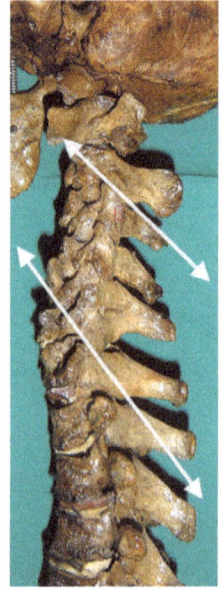

Fig. 1.4 Angulation of superior facet and hence the joint

posterior. Superior articular facet is oriented 35 degrees in sagittal plane; it increases gradually to 55° at C7 **(Fig. 1.4)**.

The lateral masses of the C7 vertebra are relatively thinner than the other cervical vertebrae. The margins of the lateral masses are defined superiorly

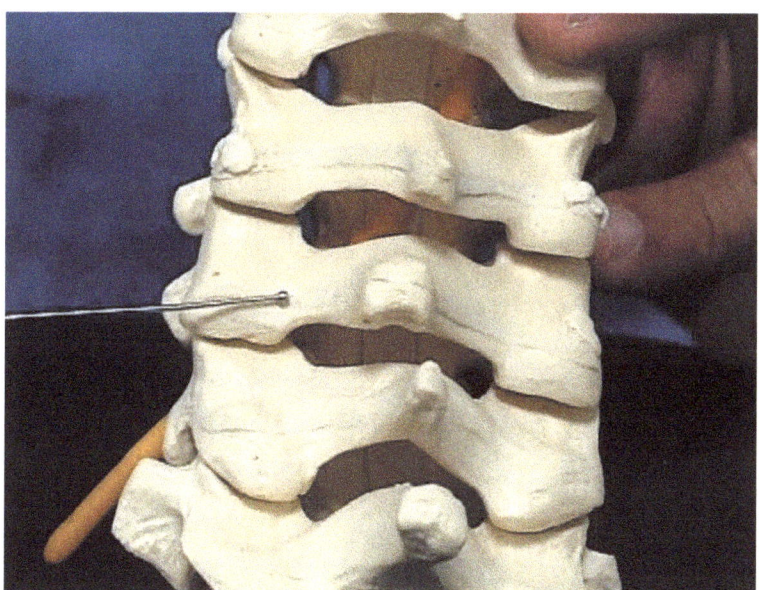

Fig. 1.5 Lateral margin of lamina

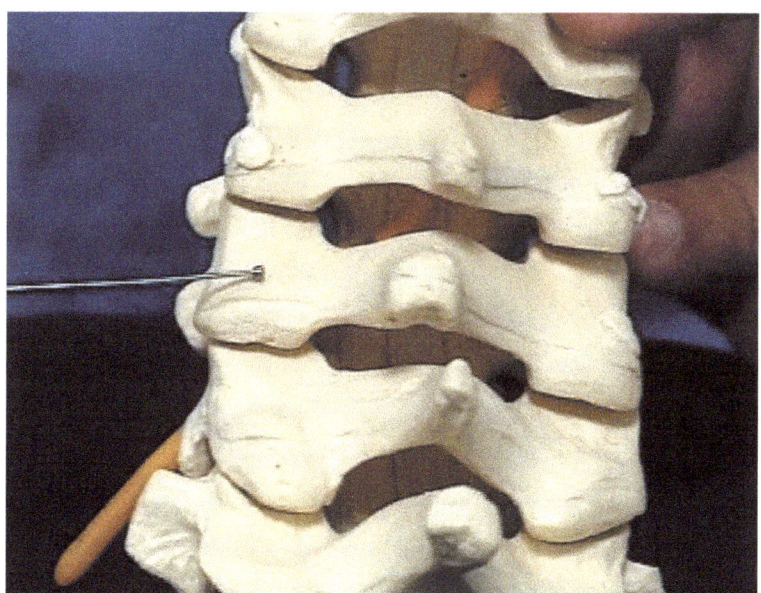

Fig. 1.6 Hillock

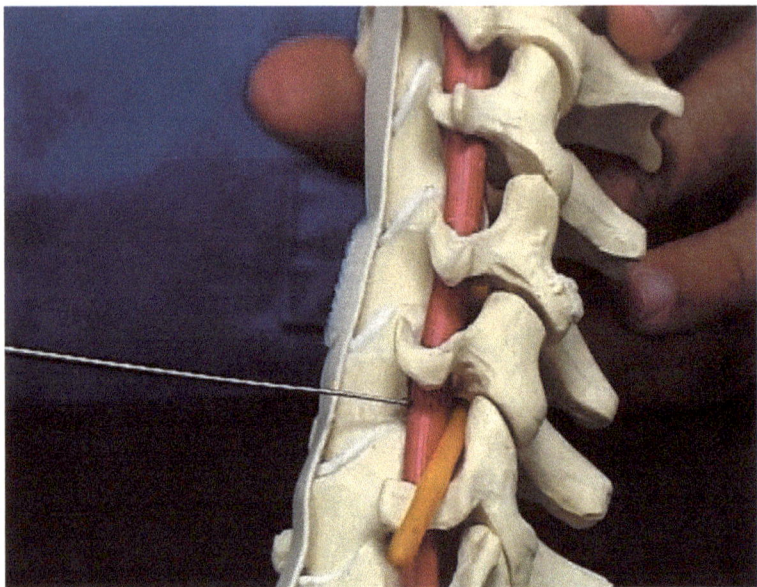

Fig. 1.7 Neurovascular structures anterior to lateral mass

and inferiorly by the facet joints, laterally by the extreme edge of the mass and medially by the lateral margin of the lamina **(Fig. 1.5)**. The center point of the mass (Hillock) is the highest point and coincides with the summit of the facet.**(Fig. 1.6)**.

The vital structures, the vertebral artery traveling through the foramen transversarium and the cranial nerve roots emerging from the spinal canal through the intervertebral foraman, are placed anterior to the lateral masses and are not seen from behind **(Fig. 1.7)**.

Chapter 2

Landmarks

The lateral mass, which is square-shaped when viewed from behind, is divided into four quadrants viz. superolateral, inferolateral, superomedial and inferomedial, using the following bony landmarks (**Fig. 2.1**):

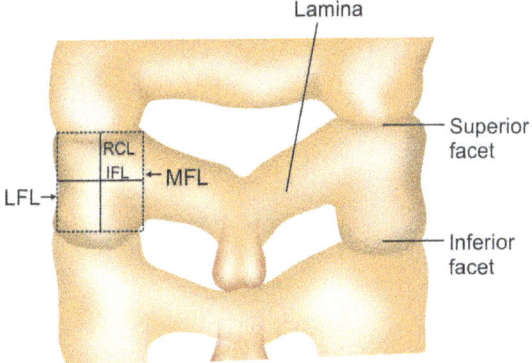

Fig. 2.1 Four quadrants

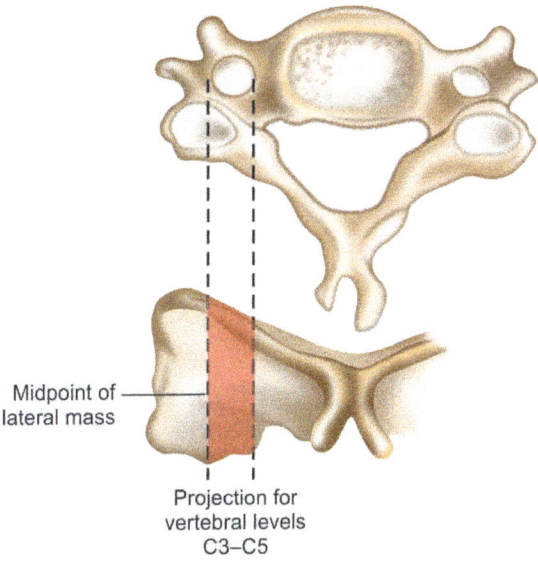

Fig. 2.2A

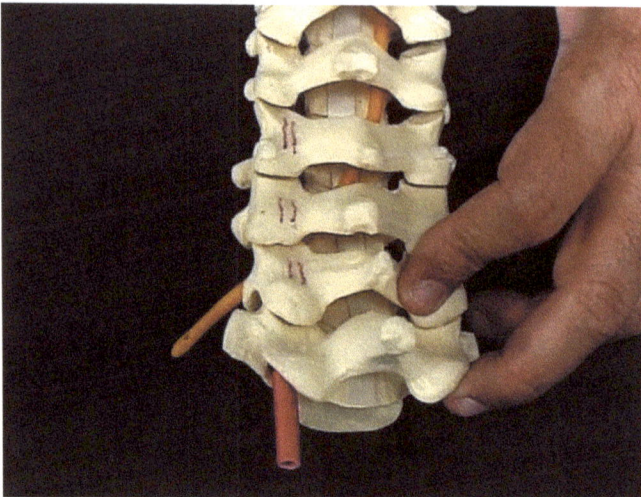

Fig. 2.2B

1. Lateral facet line (LFL), a line from one facet joint to the next facet joint along the posterolateral border of the lateral mass.
2. Medial facet line (MFL), a line from one facet joint to the next facet joint at the junction of the lamina and the lateral mass.
3. Rostrocaudal line (RCL), a line on the posterior surface of the pillar in the rostrocaudal direction dividing the mass into two vertical halves.
4. Intrafacet line (IFL), a line extending mediolaterally through the center of the mass perpendicular to the above lines. The vertebral artery courses under the superomedial and inferomedial quadrants along the medial facet line (MFL) **(Figs 2.2A and B)**.

Chapter 3

Neurovascular Structures in Relation to Lateral Mass

The cervical nerve roots, on emerging from the neural foramina, travel in a lateral, oblique, forward and downward direction from the superomedial to the inferolateral quadrant and are located anterior to the superior facet **(Figs 3.1A and B)**. During their course, the nerve roots lie dorsal to the

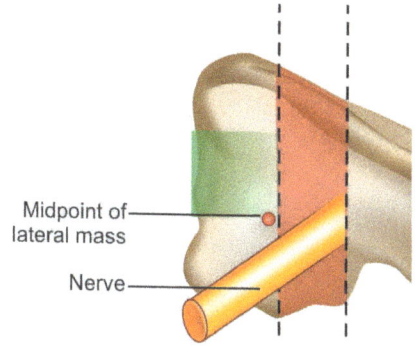

Fig. 3.1A Oblique course of the cervical nerve root

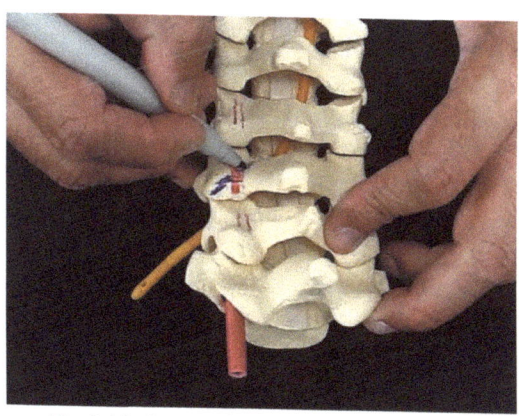

Fig. 3.1B Course of the nerve drawn with pen

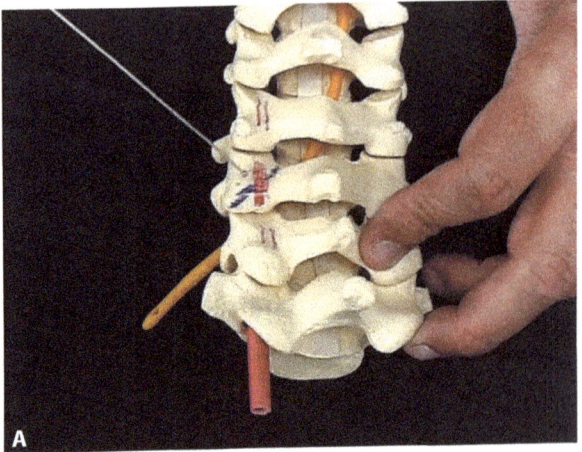

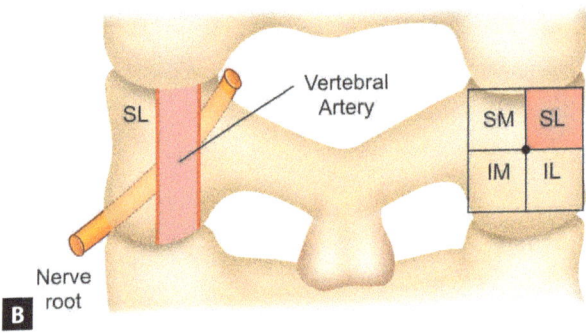

Figs 3.2A and B (A) Pointer over superolateral quadrant; (B) Safe quadrant

vertebral artery. The superolateral quadrant, under which vital neurovascular structures do not lie, is the safe quadrant and is considered ideal for the placement of lateral mass screws **(Figs 3.2A and B)**.

In addition to the basic surgical anatomy, a few critical points have to be borne in mind for proper screw placement. Cadaver studies have demonstrated variations in the measurements of the landmark lines from one lateral mass to the other and at different levels. The distance between the dorsal surface of the lateral mass peak and the underlying vertebral artery is of clinical importance. The average distance is between 9 mm and 12 mm. Hence a screw passed from a hillock straight ahead should be of 12 mm length or less to avoid vertebral artery injury **(Fig. 3.3)**. Anomalies of the vertebral artery should be kept in mind. The position of the foramen transversarium may vary in relation to each lateral mass and at different

Chapter 3: Neurovascular Structures in Relation to Lateral Mass

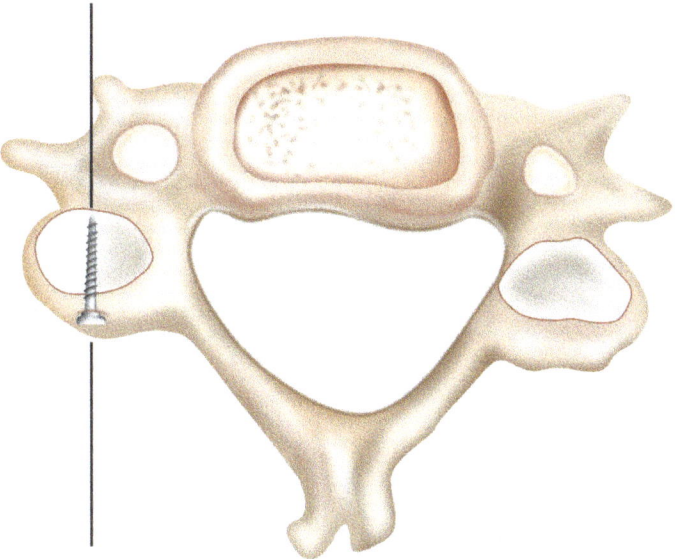

Fig. 3.3 Distance between hillock and foramen transversarium

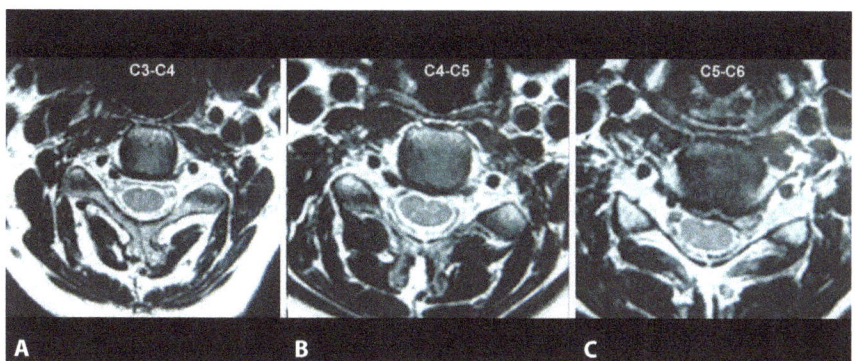

Figs 3.4A to C MRI pictures demonstrating vertebral artery position

levels. Axial cuts of the CT and MR scans will help in determining that of the exact lateral angulation required to enable safe placement of the screws **(Figs 3.4A to C)**. The lateral masses are regularly oval in the axial cut and squarish dome shaped in the posterior. This knowledge is important in selecting the entry point of the screw to gain maximum purchase of the lateral mass.

CRITICAL POINTS

1. The average distance between the dorsal surface of the lateral mass peak and the vertebral artery is between 9 mm and 12 mm. Hence a screw passed from the hillock should be of 12 mm or less to avoid injury to the artery if directed straight ahead.
2. The position of foramen transversarium varies anatomically. Hence, a preoperative CT assessment is essential to judge the lateral angulation of screw trajectory.
3. The lateral masses are irregularly oval in the axial cut and squarish dome shaped posteriorly. This knowledge is important in selecting the entry point to get the maximum purchase of screw in the mass.

Chapter 4

Standard Screw Trajectories

There are many trajectories described in the literature regarding screw placement. The site of entry is either at the center or medial to the center of the lateral mass in order to gain the maximum purchase. Universally, each school has advocated placing the screws in the superolateral quadrant. However, the lateral angulation varies from 10° to 30° and the direction of the screws in the sagittal plane varies from the perpendicular to the long axis of the spine (straight ahead) to 40° cephalad (parallel to facet joints).

SCREW TRAJECTORIES AND CRITICAL POINTS

- The more medial and cephalad the trajectory, the more likely it is for nerve root injury to occur.
- Risks of facet joints and incorporation of the neighboring motion segment occur when the screws were directed strictly anterior.
- Various school of trajectories are enumerated.

School	Site of entry	Sagittal plane angulation	Lateral angulation
Roy Camille	Center	Straight ahead (perpendicular)	10°
Magerl	1–2 mm medial and rostral	40° cephalad and parallel to facet joints	25°
An, Trynalis, Haid	1 mm medial	15° cephalad	20°–30°
	1 mm medial	10°–20° cephalad	30°
Anderson	1 mm medial	Parallel to facet joints	10°
Cooper	1 mm medial	Perpendicular to long axis of spine	10°

Hence, a screw directed superiorly and laterally from the hillock will be placed in the superolateral quadrant thus avoiding the neurovascular structures.

Magerl Technique

Entry point: Just superior and medial to the hillock or the midpoint (**Fig. 4.1**).

Section 1: Basics

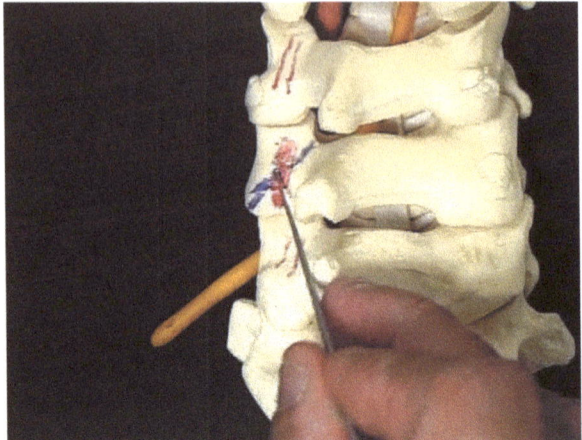

Fig. 4.1 Magerl entry point

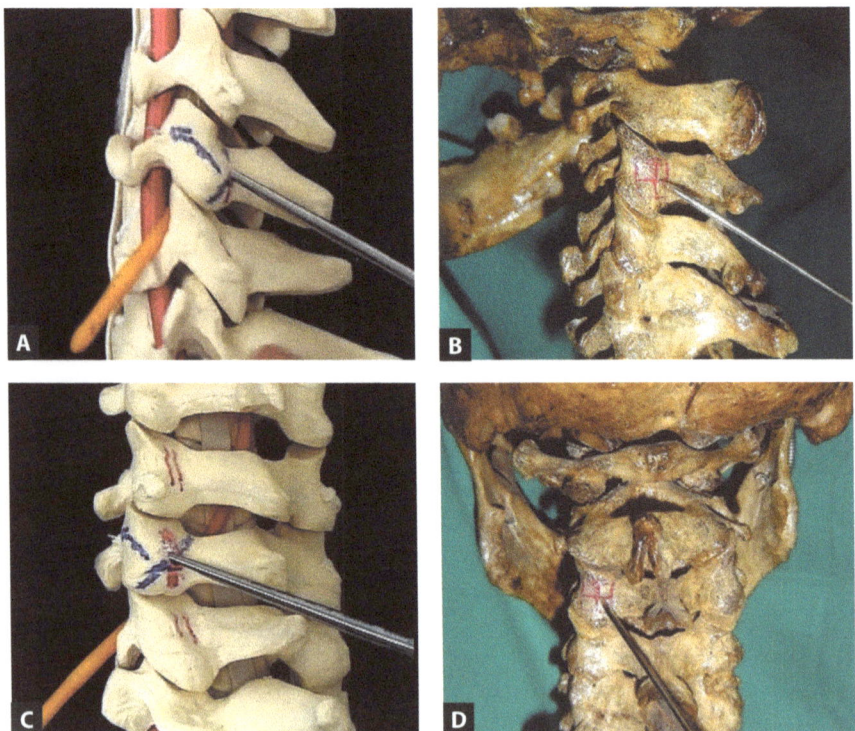

Figs 4.2A to D (A and B) Superiorly directed; (C and D) Laterally directed

Chapter 4: Standard Screw Trajectories   15

Probing from this entry point is directed superiorly 40°—parallel to facet joint **(Figs 4.2A and B)** and laterally 25° **(Figs 4.2C and D)** until the distal cortex is pierced. The glow end of the probe usually come close to the spinous process of the inferior spine.

Screws placed in this way avoid neurovascular structures anteriorly **(Figs 4.3A and B)**.

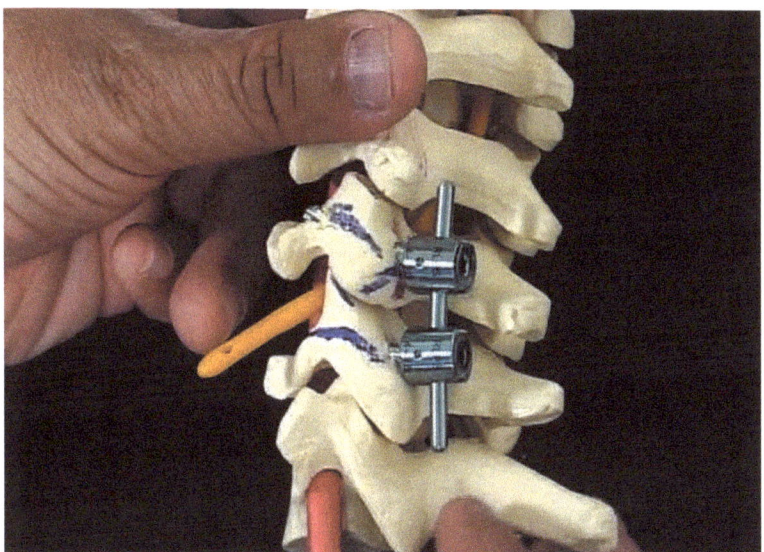

Fig. 4.3A Lateral mass fixation with bicortical screws

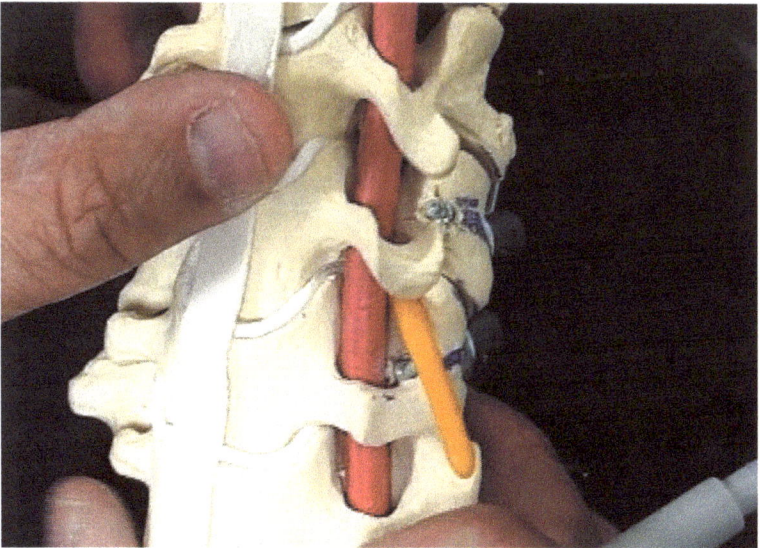

Figs 4.3B Note the distal end of screws not violating the neurovascular structures

Section 2

Surgical Techniques

Chapter 5

Positioning the Patient

After endotracheal general anesthesia using a flexometallic tube **(Fig. 5.1)**, a Mayfield three pin fixator is fixed to the skull firmly **(Fig. 5.2)**. Bladder should be catheterized and the lower limbs need to be supported with TED stockings or intermittent compressors **(Fig. 5.3)**.

Patient should then be gently turned without disturbing the cervical spine **(Fig. 5.4)** and is positioned prone over a pair of bolsters. The head clamp is then fixed to the table. The neck is well exposed and skin folds avoided **(Figs 5.5A and B)**. Endotracheal tube should be fixed to the clamp so that it is well secured **(Fig. 5.6)**.

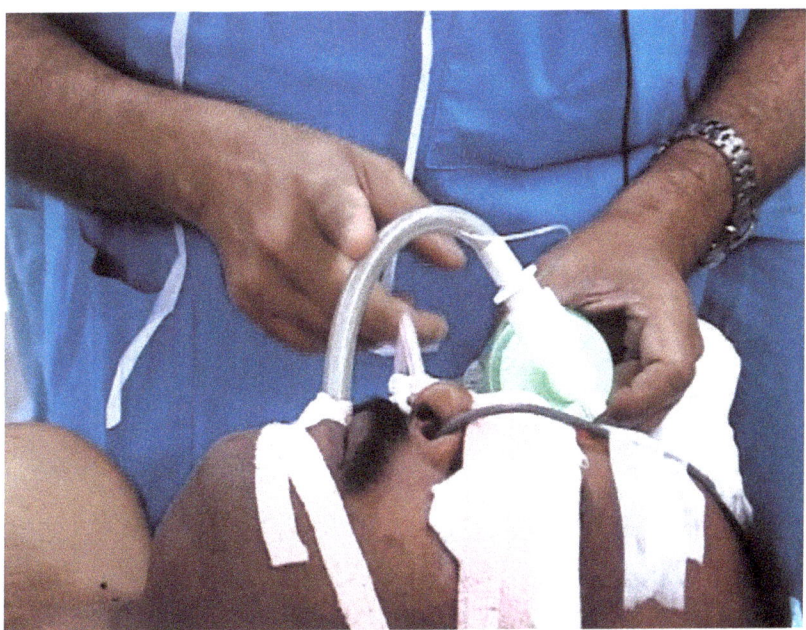

Fig. 5.1 Flexometallic endotracheal tube

20 Section 2: Surgical Techniques

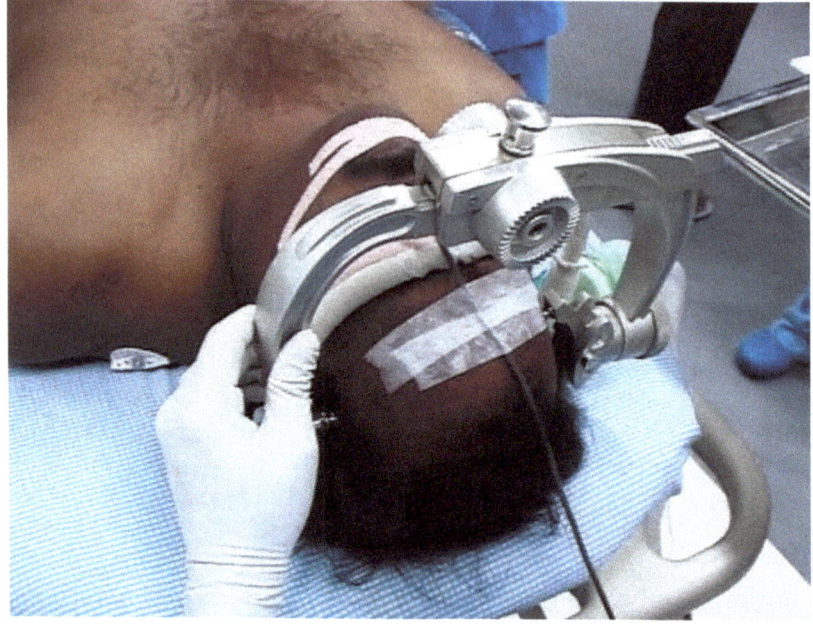

Fig. 5.2 Mayfield three pin head clamp

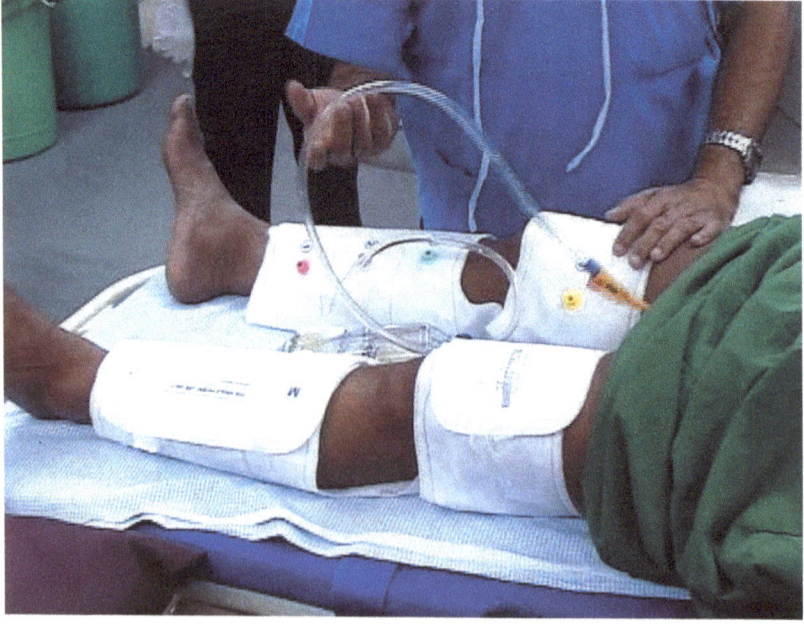

Fig. 5.3 Bladder catheter and intermittent compressor

Chapter 5: Positioning the Patient 21

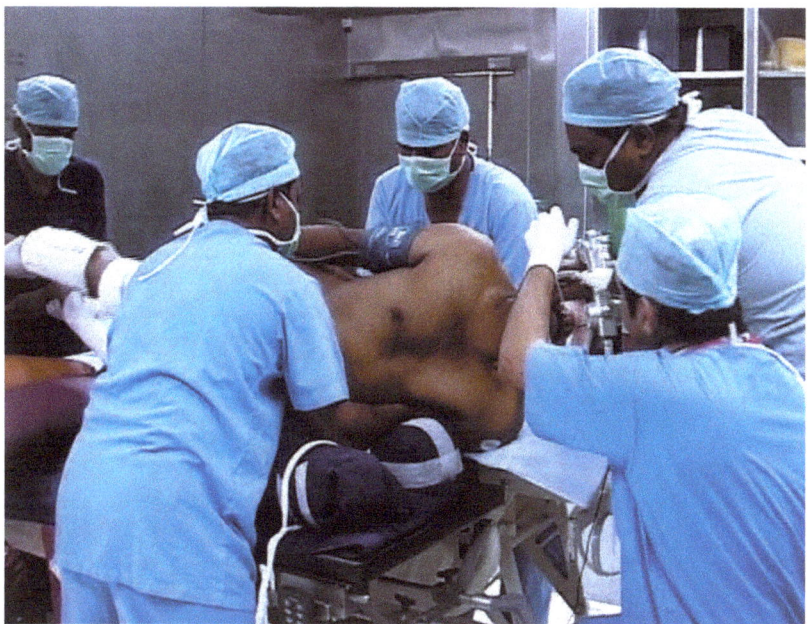

Fig. 5.4 Judicious turning of the patient. Note the lead surgeon at the head end

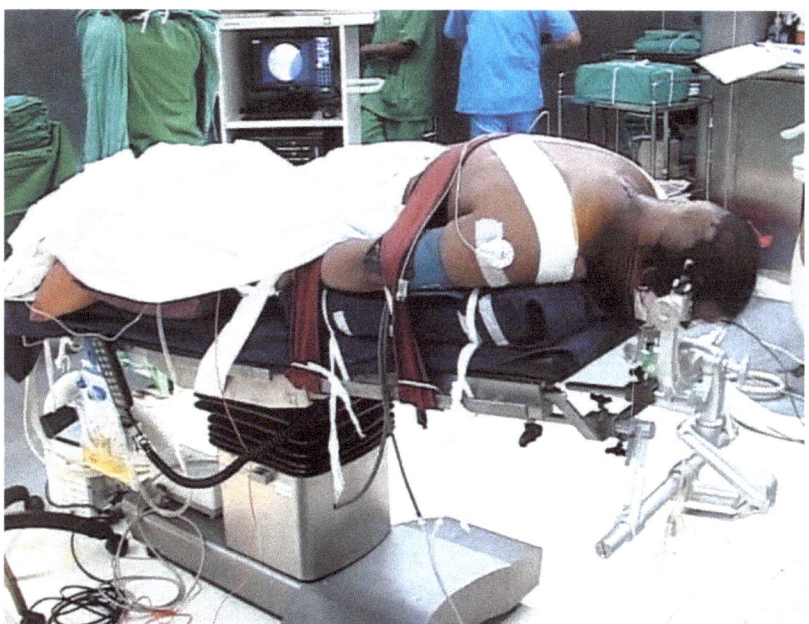

Fig. 5.5A Classical prone position on the table

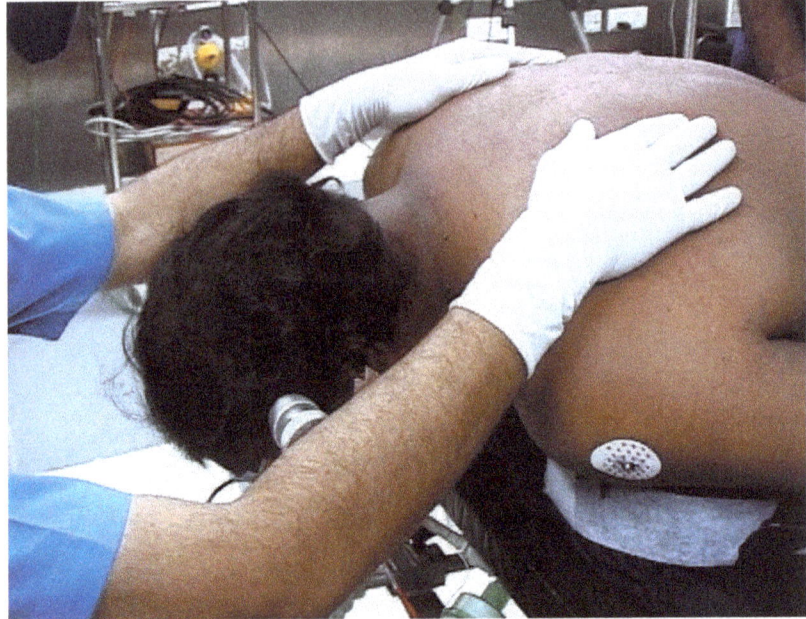

Fig. 5.5B Avoid neck skin folding

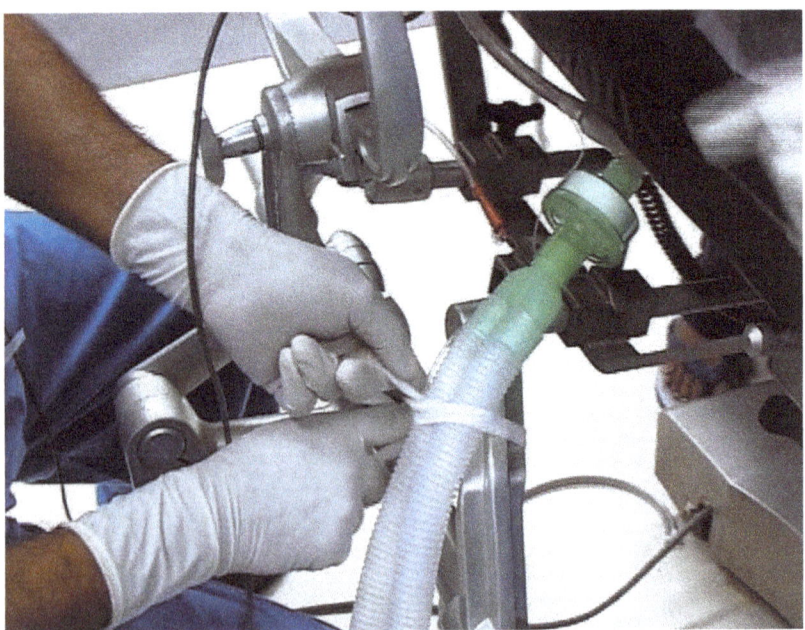

Fig. 5.6 Secure the endotracheal tube

Chapter 6

Exposure

Step 1: A midline incision is made from occipital protuberance to T1 spinous process which can be extended below to expose one level above and below the level of interest. Larger incisions always give good exposure of the spine **(Fig. 6.1)**. A mixture of Lignocaine and adrenaline be infiltrated subcutaneously below the incision and also in the paraspinal muscles both sides. This effectively reduce the blood loss and increases the comfort. Anesthetists discussion is needed routinely in all patients.

We always check the images of cervical spine before draping with an image intensifier **(Fig. 6.2)**. This is to make minimal adjustments in cervical spine position if needed in special situations.

I insist my technicians to mark the position of the image intensifier wheels to avoid chaotic changes when imaging is required in the middle

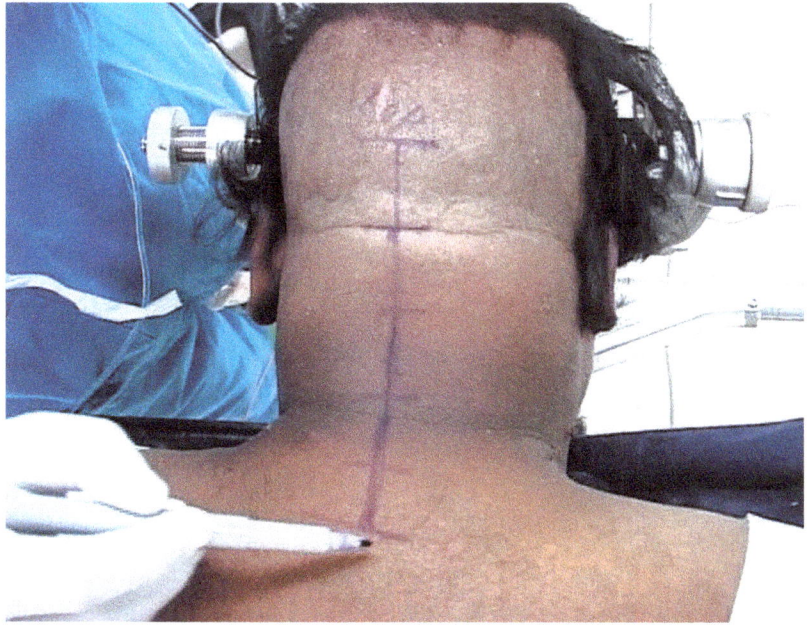

Fig. 6.1 Midline skin mark

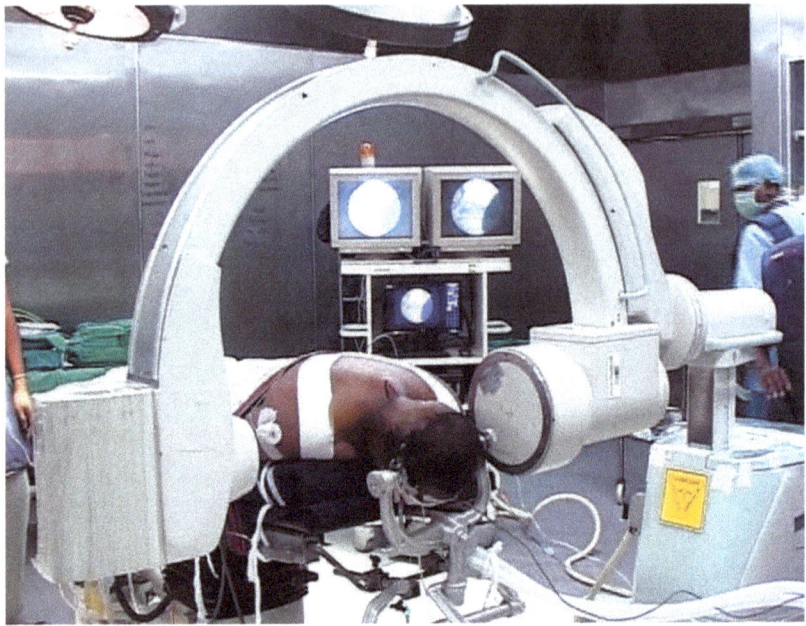

Fig. 6.2 Peroperative imaging to assess the alignment of cervical spine

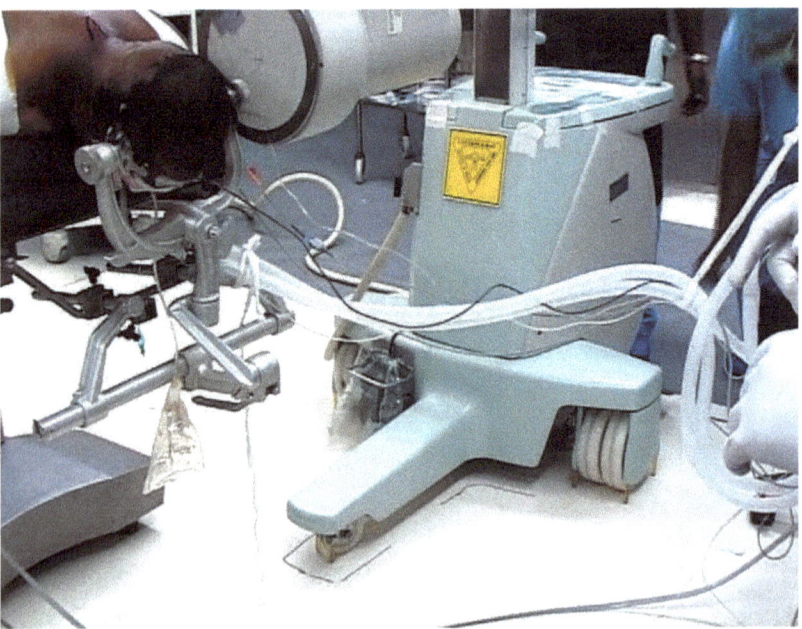

Fig. 6.3 Marking the base of image intensifier on the floor

of the surgery. This will reduce over exposure to radiation to a large extent **(Fig. 6.3)**.

Step 2: The skin and subcutaneous tissue are incised up to the spinous processes **(Figs 6.4A and B)**. Paraspinal muscles are separated subperiosteally from spinous process, lamina and the entire lateral mass is exposed to its lateral border **(Figs 6.5A and B)**. Care should be taken to preserve the ligaments and the facet joints.

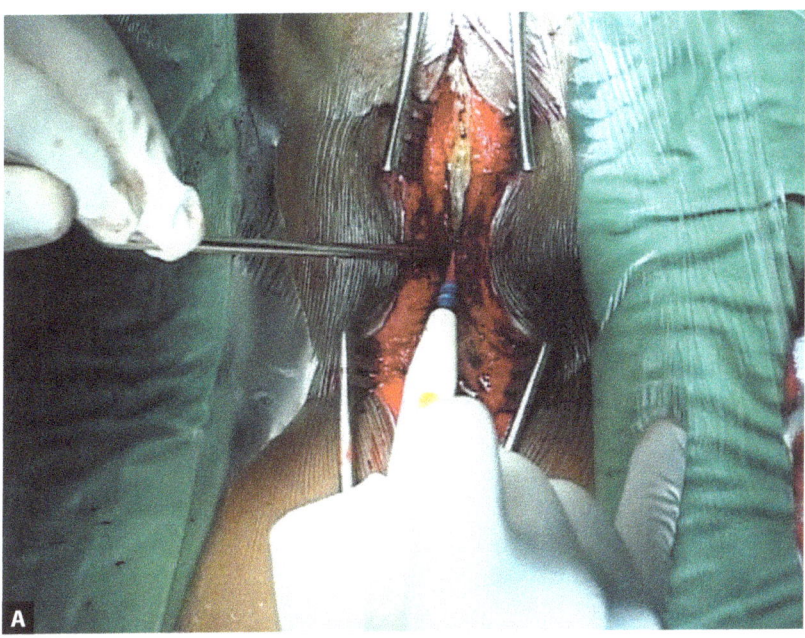

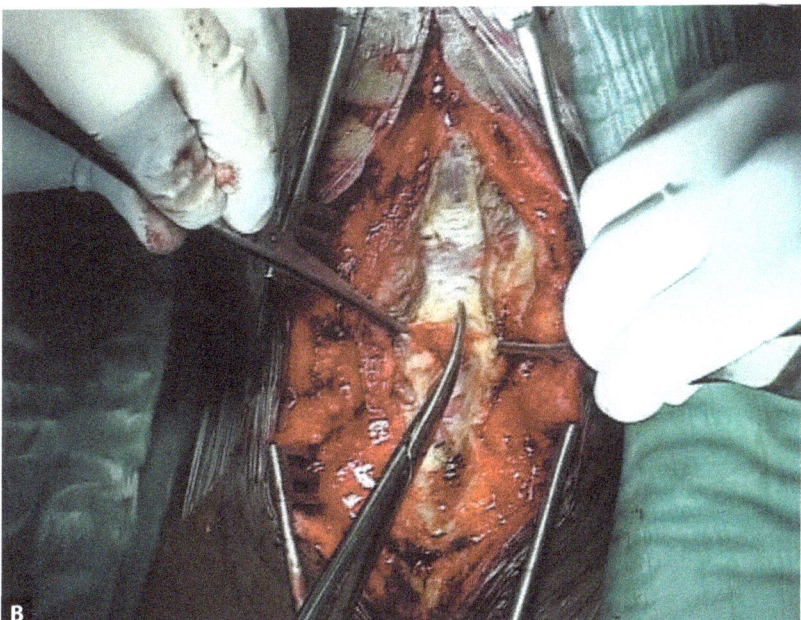

Figs 6.4A and B (A) Monopolar cautery cut over the midline; (B) Midline nuchal fascia cut with scissors

26 Section 2: Surgical Techniques

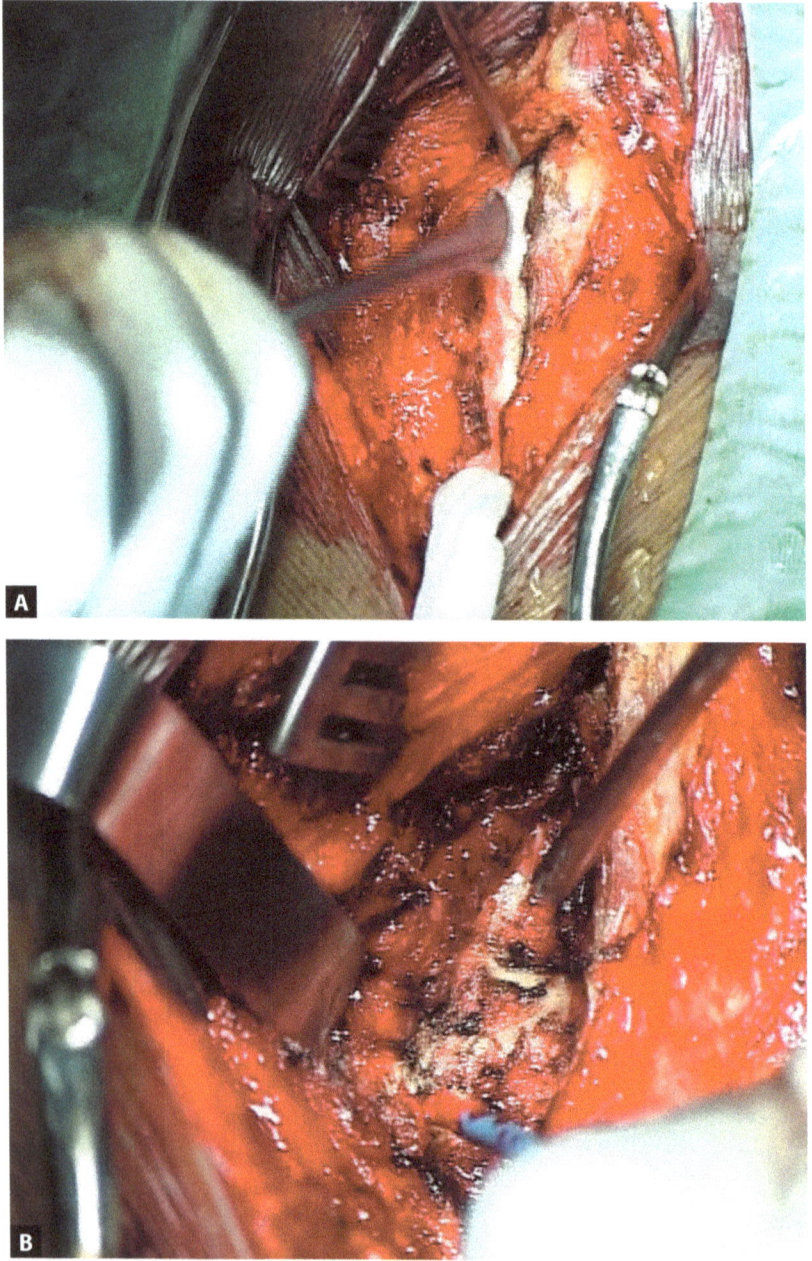

Figs 6.5A and B (A) Paraspinal muscles retracted laterally; (B) Lateral mass exposed up to the lateral border

Step 3: Each lateral mass is inspected carefully on both sides **(Fig. 6.6)**. This is very important particularly in trauma patients. In some patients jumped superior facets or fractured fragments can be seen **(Figs 6.6A to C)**.

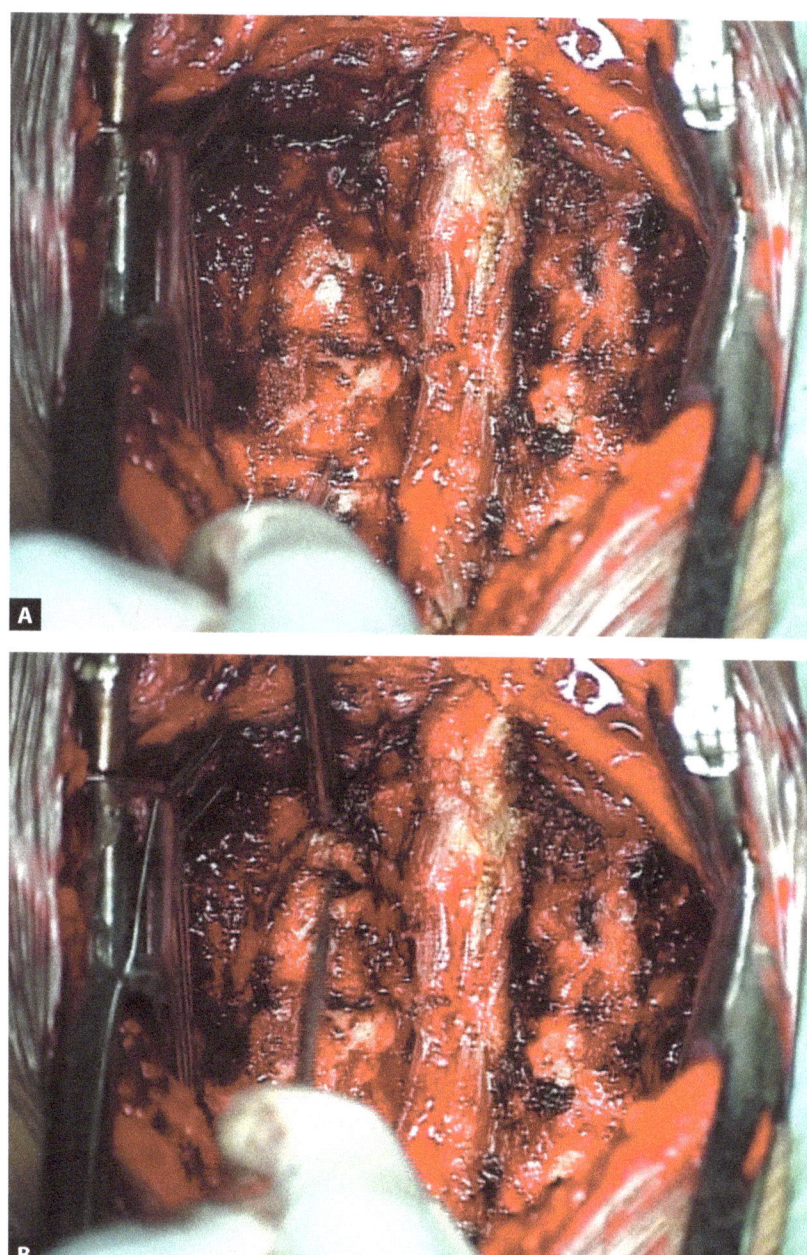

Figs 6.6A and B (A) Lateral masses on both sides exposed up to their border; (B) Facet joint inspection

Identify and feel the lateral border of the lateral mass (LM) **(Fig. 6.7A)**, superiorly facet joint **(Fig. 6.7B)**, inferiorly the inferior facet **(Fig. 6.7C)** and medially the shallow region the lamina meets the LM **(Fig. 6.7D)**.

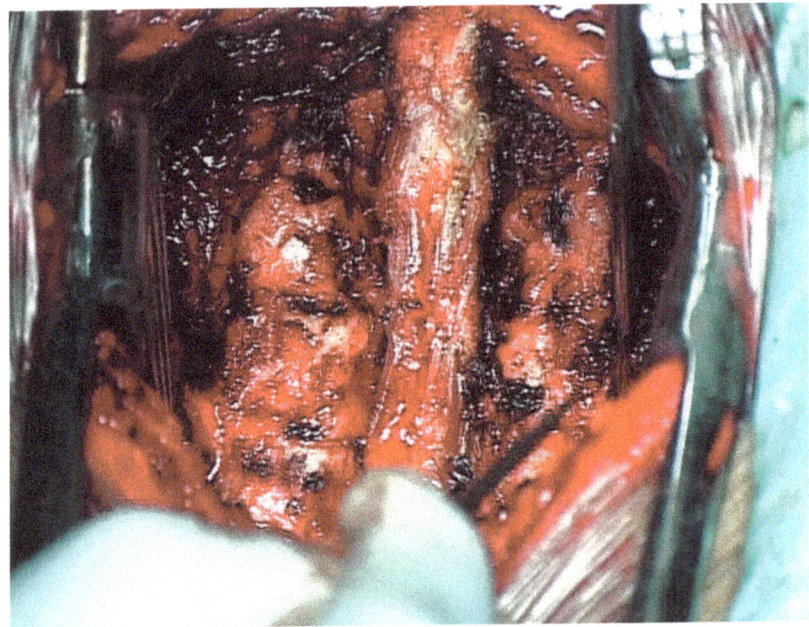

Fig. 6.6C Opposite site facet joint inspection

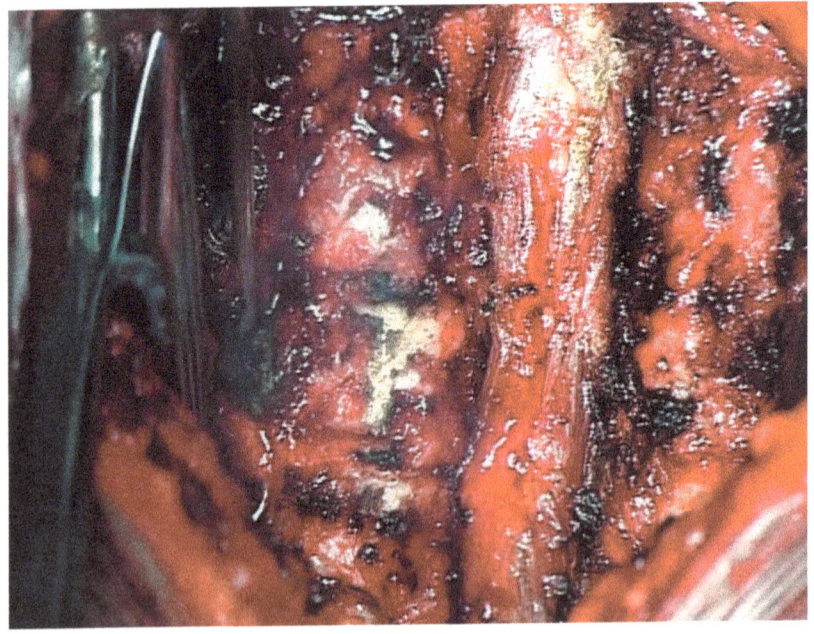

Fig. 6.7A Lateral border marked

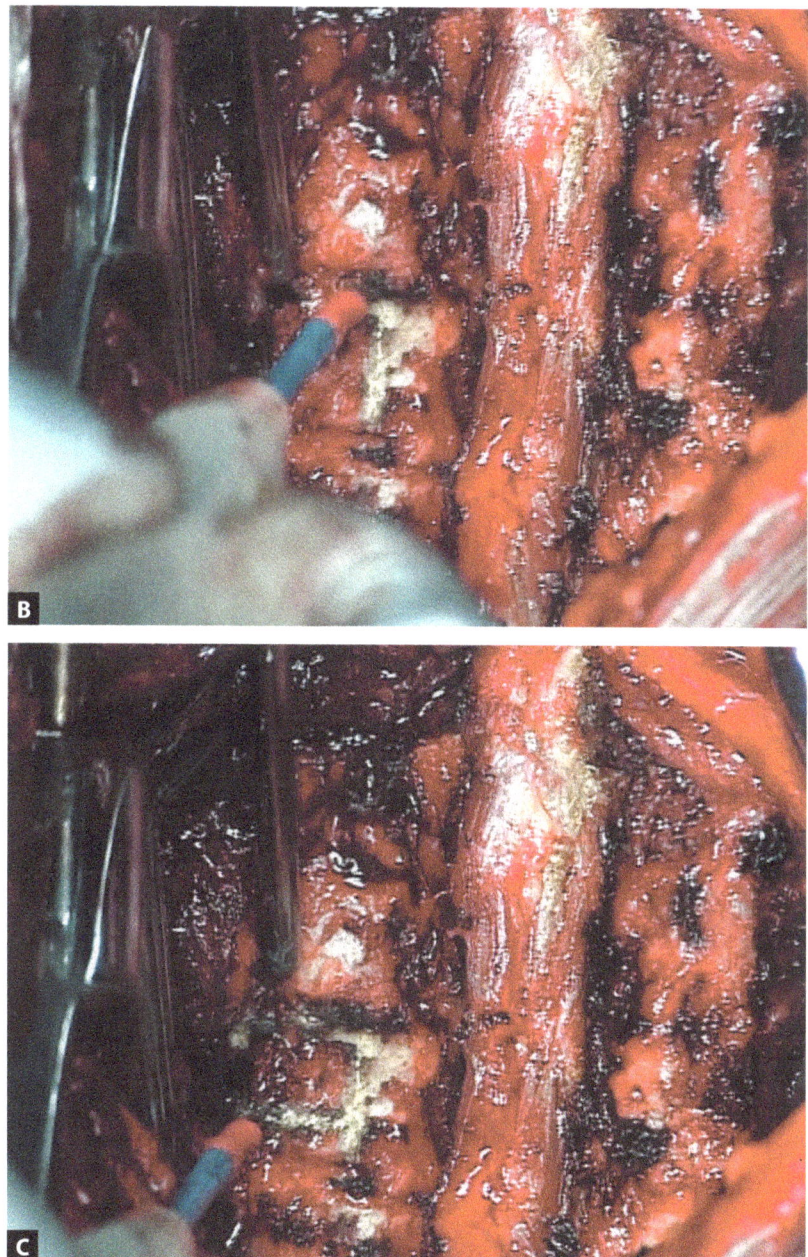

Figs 6.7B and C (B) Superior facet joint identified and superior border marked; (C) Inferior facet identified and inferior border marked

Mark the borders with a monopolar cautery and then draw the four quadrants **(Fig. 6.8)**. The midpoint of all quadrants the central point, corresponds to the highest point of the lateral mass is now identified **(Fig. 6.9)**.

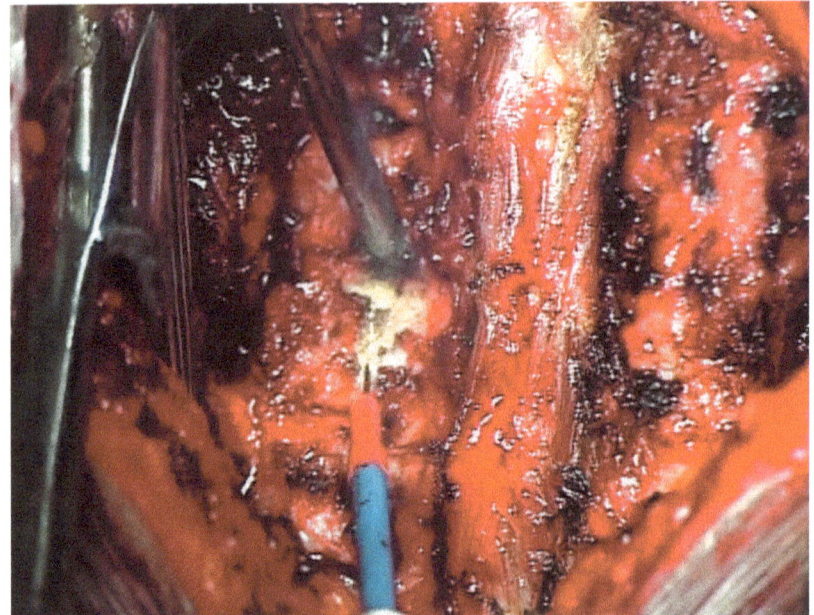

Fig. 6.7D Medial border marked

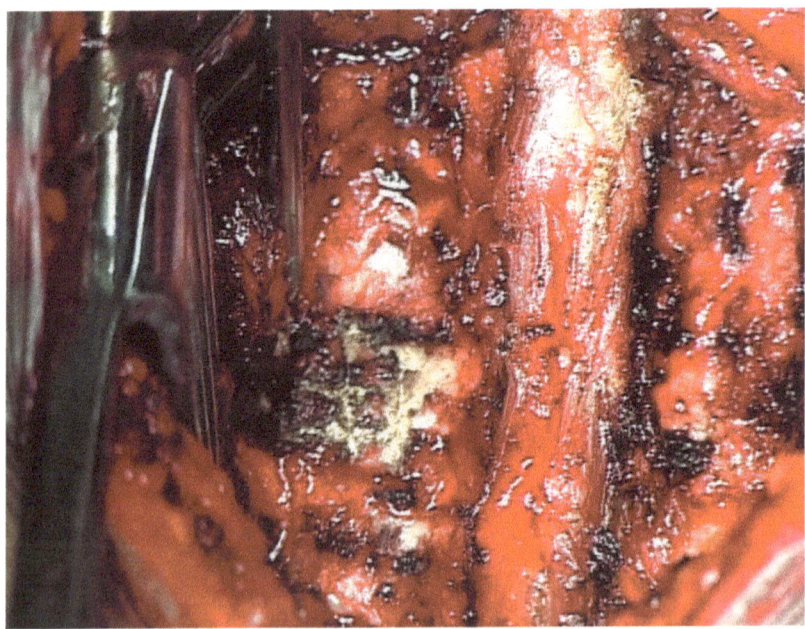

Fig. 6.8 All four quadrants marked with monopolar cautery

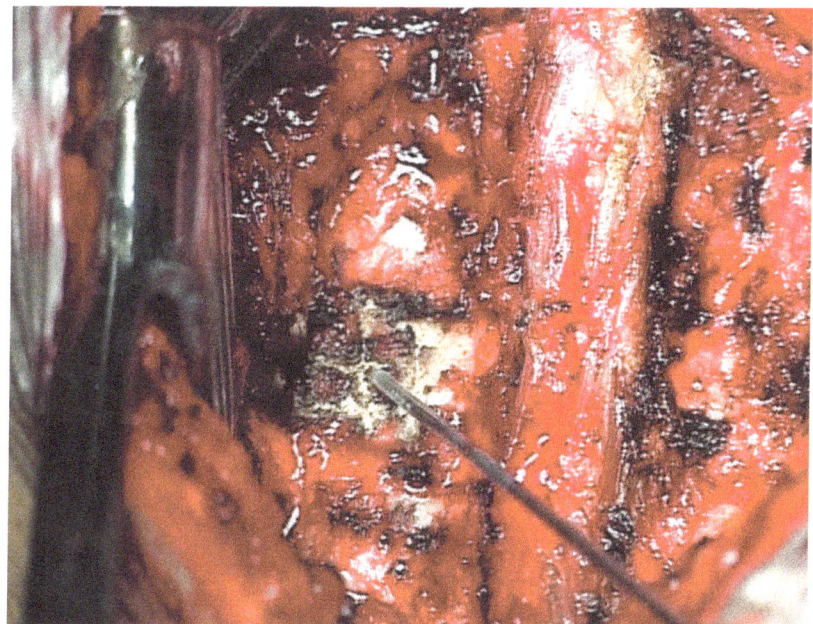

Fig. 6.9 Center point identified which corresponds to the hillock commonly

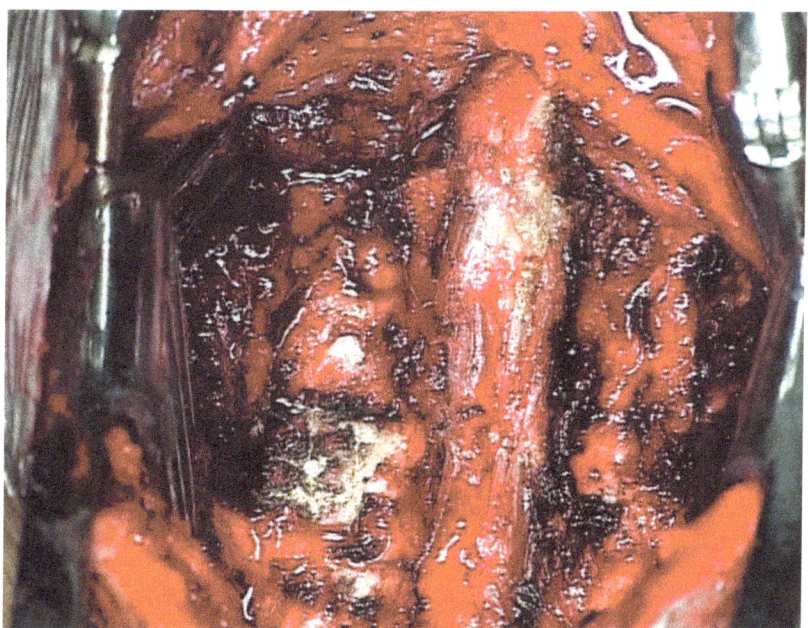

Fig. 6.10 Screw entry point marked with monopolar cautery

The screw entry point is selected 1 mm medial and superior to the center is usually selected **(Fig. 6.10)**. This is to ensure good purchase of the screw in LM. Some times surgeons may have to adjust and select the best entry point over the hillock. If not properly done the screws may slip and damage the LM.

Chapter 7

Drilling

Step 1: Using a 2.7 mm diameter diamond drill bit the outer cortex of the entry point is pierced gently at slow speed and then the drill is angled 25° laterally and 40° rostrally into the eventual trajectory of screw placement in the supralateral quadrant of the lateral mass **(Fig. 7.1)**.

Step 2: Steady and precise drilling is performed until the inner cortex is pierced, which will be felt by a 'give way' sensation. Bicortical purchase is essential for good fixation **(Fig. 7.2)**. I personally do not recommend hand drills. They have less control and can slip out more often and the cervical movement during the procedure look dangerous and uncomfortable. These technical hazards are less reported and taught. A good motorized mini drill system with long handle is ideal and recommended.

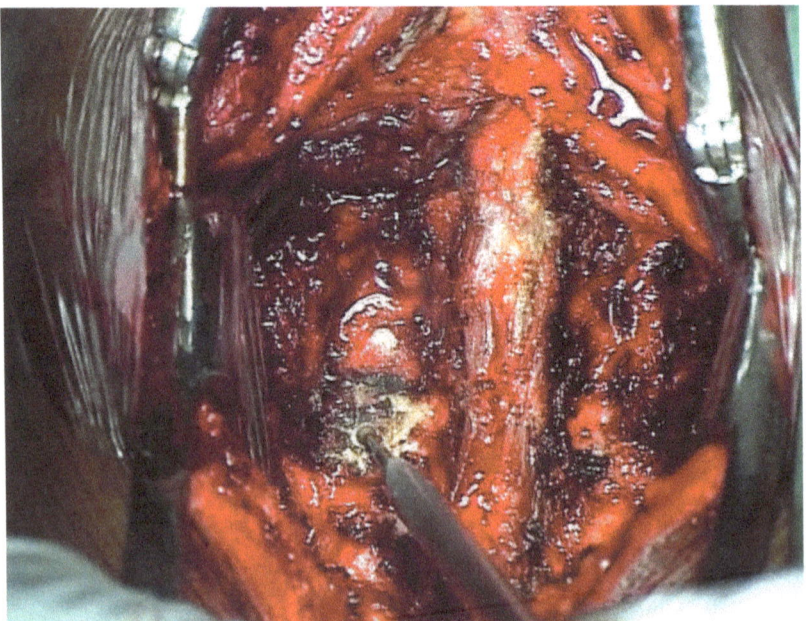

Fig. 7.1 Drilling the outer cortex using diamond burr

Chapter 7: Drilling 33

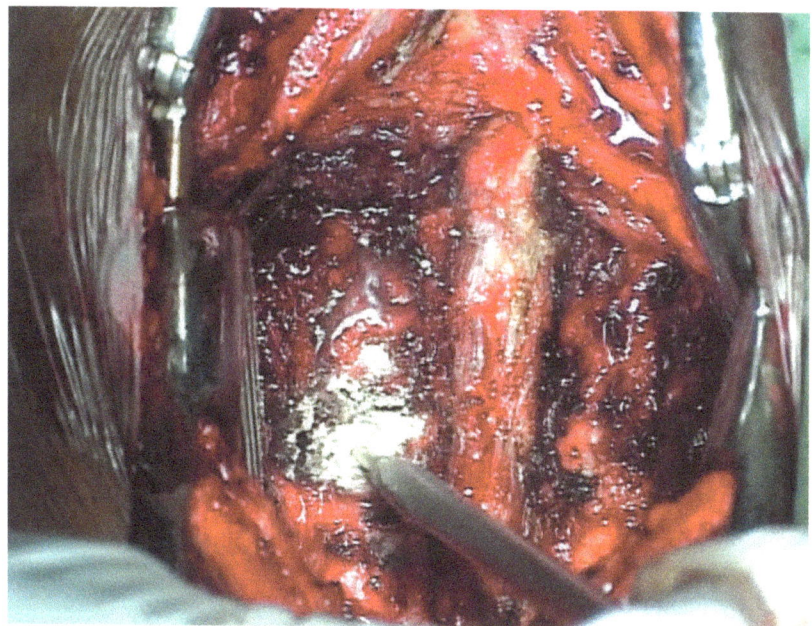

Fig. 7.2 Advancing the drill gently until the inner cortex is pierced

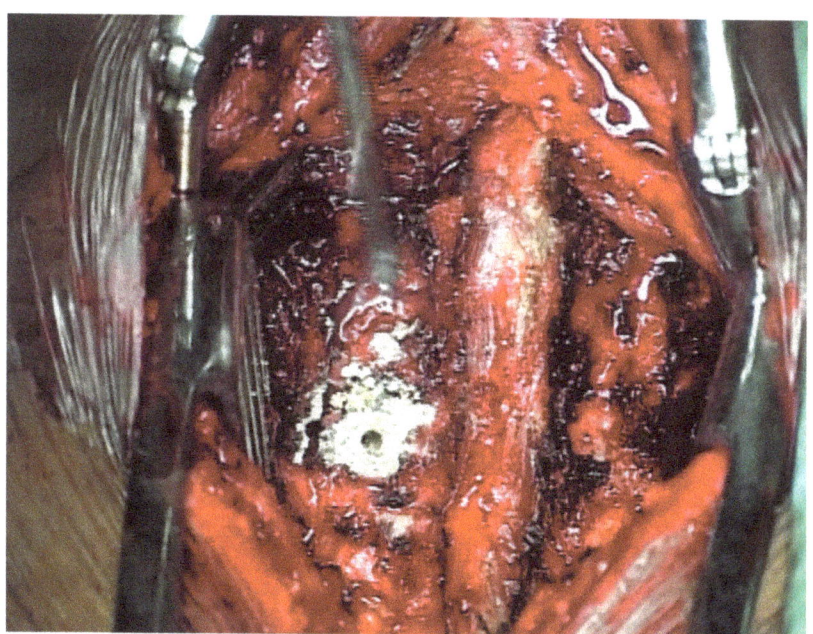

Fig. 7.3 Drill hole site

Section 2: Surgical Techniques

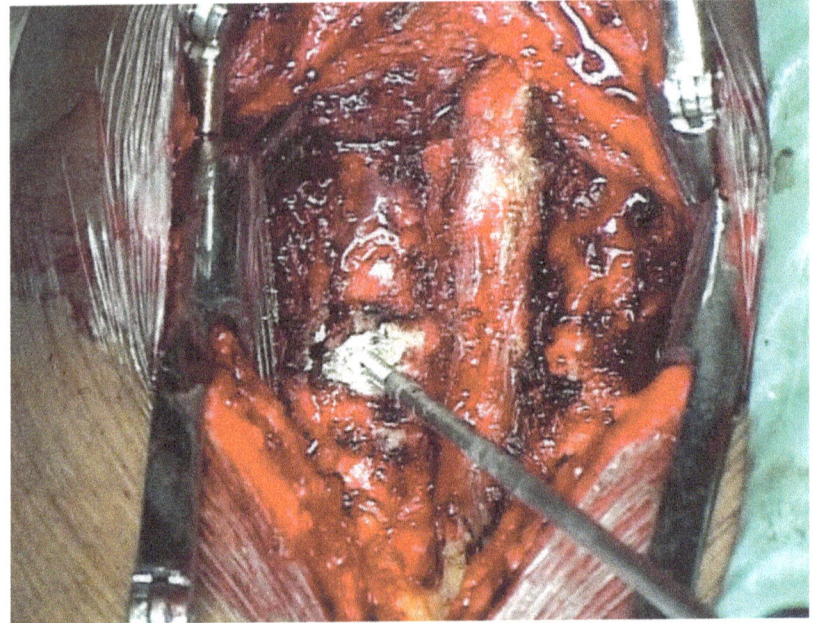

Fig. 7.4 Tapping gently

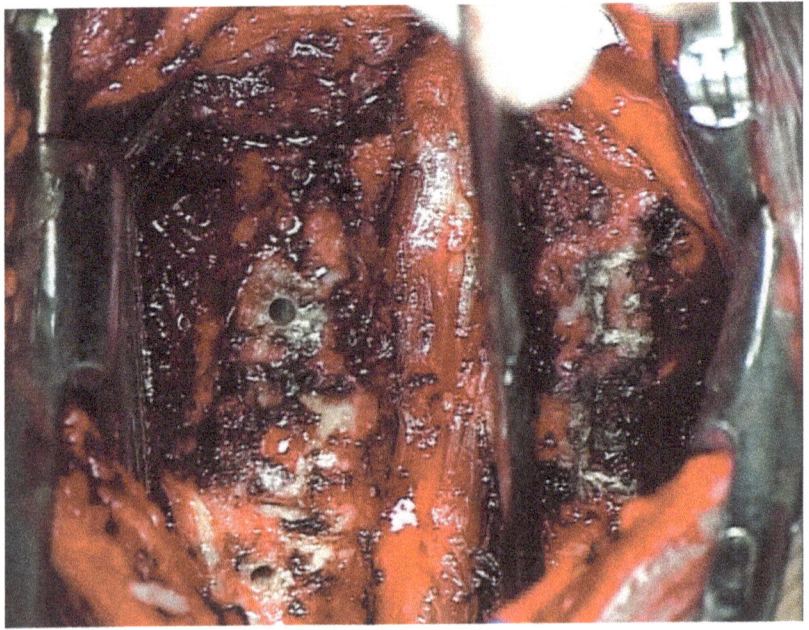

Fig. 7.5 Other lateral mass drill holes made

Chapter 7: Drilling 35

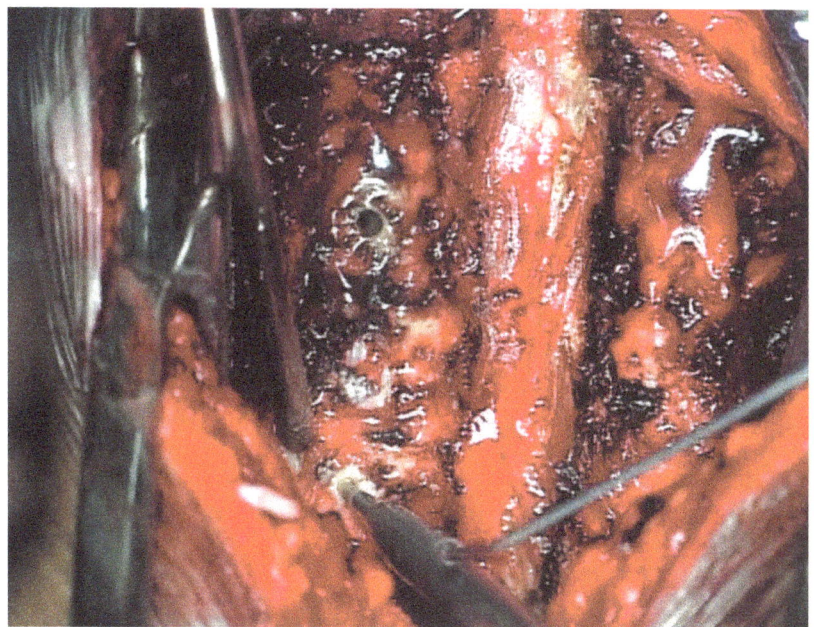

Fig. 7.6 Saline irrigation while drilling

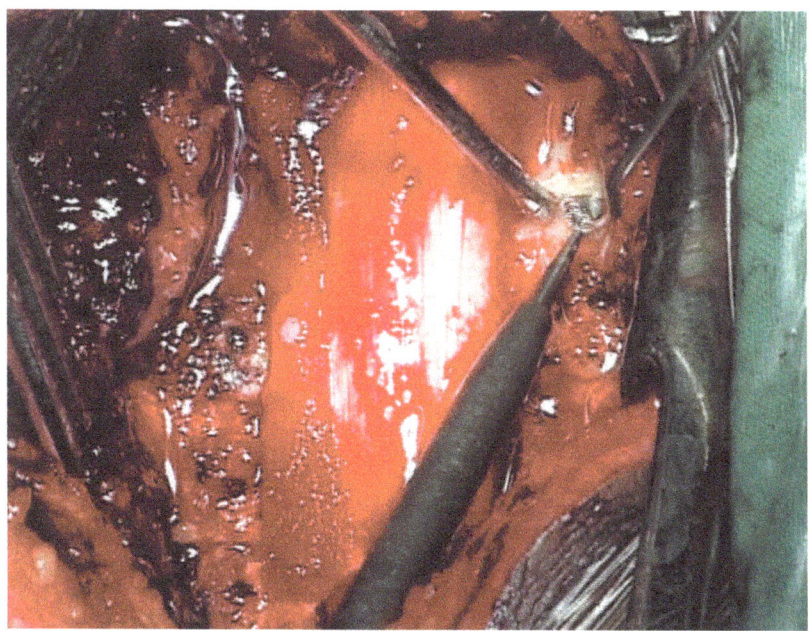

Fig. 7.7 Graft bed preparation of the facet joint

Bone wax can be used to arrest the blood ooze from the drilled hole site. **(Fig. 7.3)**.

Step 3: Appropriate tap is used to tap the outer cortex **(Fig. 7.4)**.

Like this way all lateral masses are drilled on the same side first **(Fig. 7.5)** and then on the opposite side for screw placements later **(Fig. 7.6)**. I usually complete posterior decompression (Laminectomy) before placing the screws.

Step 4: At C7 and T1 the entry point is selected just lateral to the center of lateral mass, 1 mm to caudal to the facet joint. Trajectory of drilling will be 25° to 30° medial to the sagittal plane and parallel to upper end plate. This is basically the pedicular screws and not lateral mass screws. It is mentioned here to complete the subject.

Step 5: Facet joints can be decorticated for fusion bed preparation **(Fig. 7.7)**.

Chapter 8

Instrumentation

Step 1: Polyaxial screws of appropriate length (14 mm–18 mm) are then inserted in the lateral masses one by one without producing abnormal torques while placing **(Figs 8.1A to D)**.

Fusion bed at facet joint is now packed with cancellous and cortical bones harvested from iliac crest. This will augment fusion **(Fig. 8.2)**.

Step 2: Tapes or flexible measurement rods are used to prepare the length and contour of the rod needed **(Fig. 8.3)**. Rods are cut to required lengths and bent for lordosis especially in 3 vertebrae fixation. Trial placement of rods are done before securing finally **(Fig. 8.4)** and then secured to the screws with check nuts **(Figs 8.5A to D)**. Over tightening should be avoided.

Step 3: Hemostasis is secured well. Gelforms placed over the dura **(Fig. 8.6)**. A drain is placed in the epidural space and brought out through the paraspinal

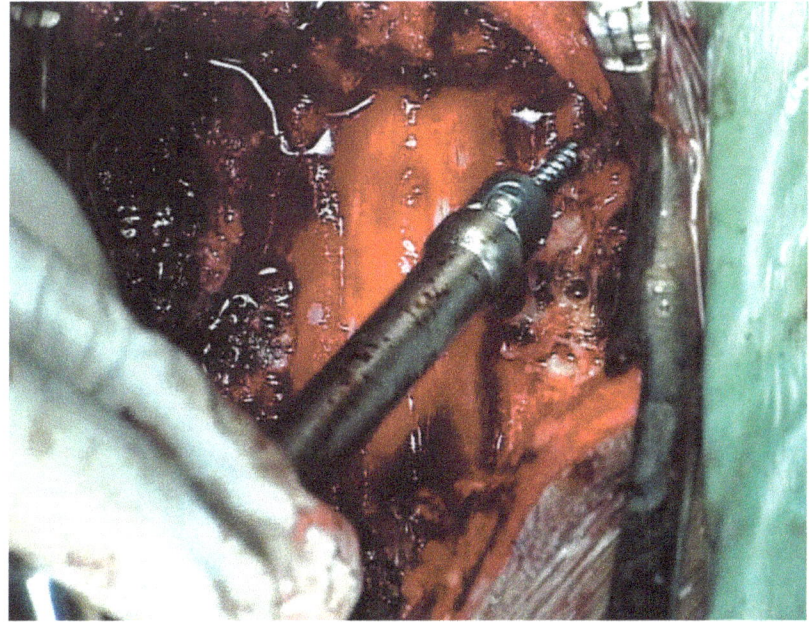

Fig. 8.1A Polyaxial screw placement at the superior most lateral mass

38 Section 2: Surgical Techniques

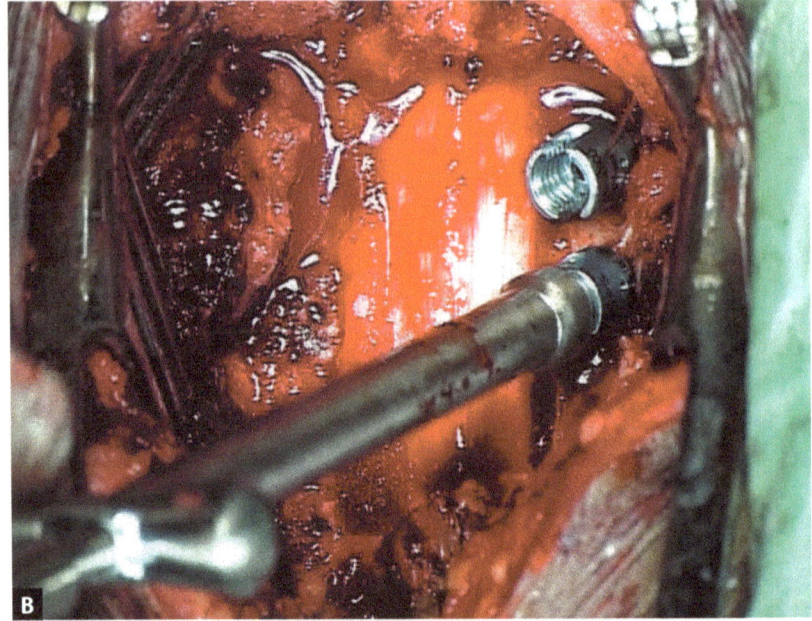

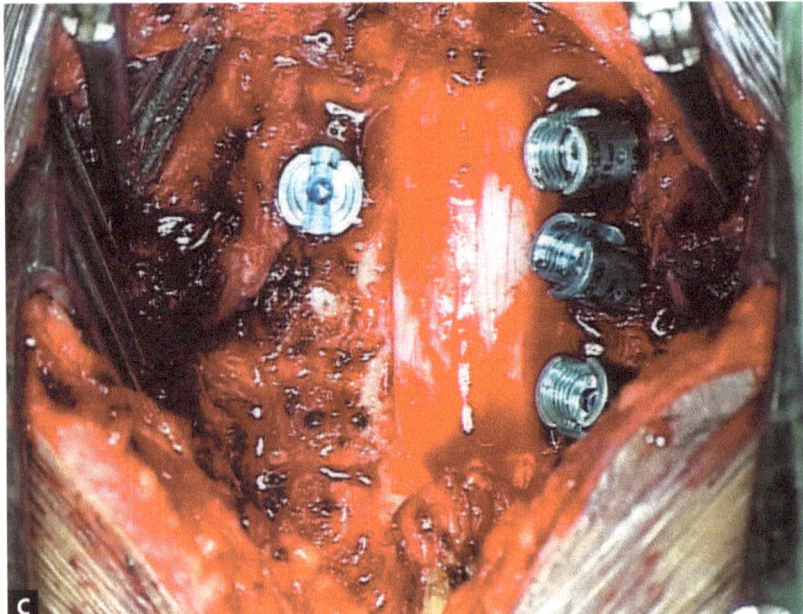

Figs 8.1B and C (B) Next screw placement just inferior to the superior site; (C) Opposite side superior screw placed

muscle by separate wound lateral to the incision. The fascia covering the paraspinal muscles are approximated at the midline with absorbable suture material. Avoid paraspinal muscles included in the suture. Subcutaneous

Chapter 8: Instrumentation 39

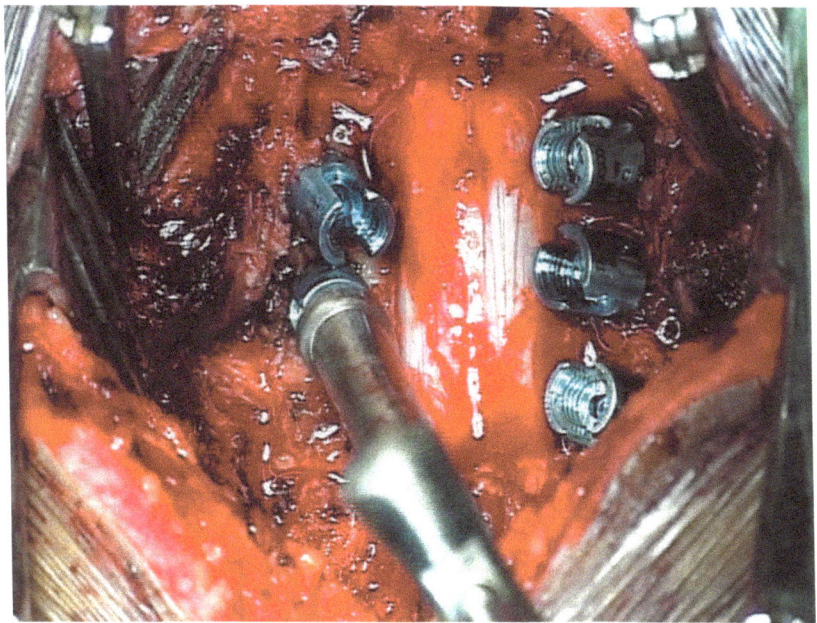

Fig. 8.1D Opposite side next screw placement just inferior to the superior site

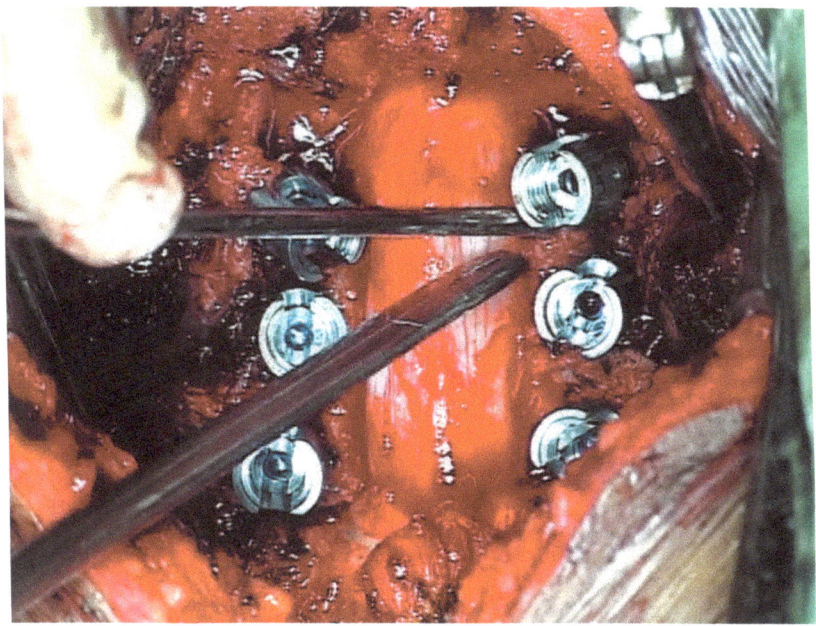

Fig. 8.2 Facet joint grafting

40 Section 2: Surgical Techniques

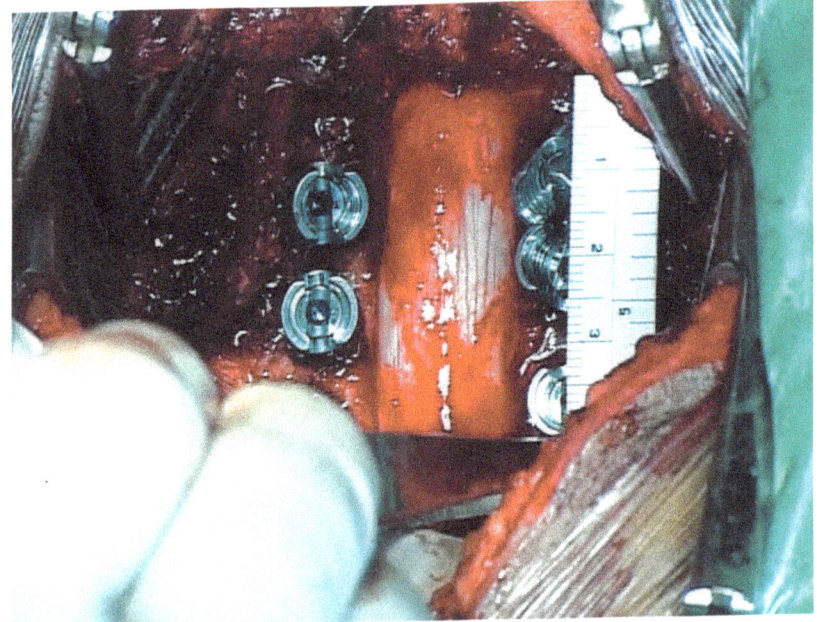

Fig. 8.3 Measuring length for appropriate rod

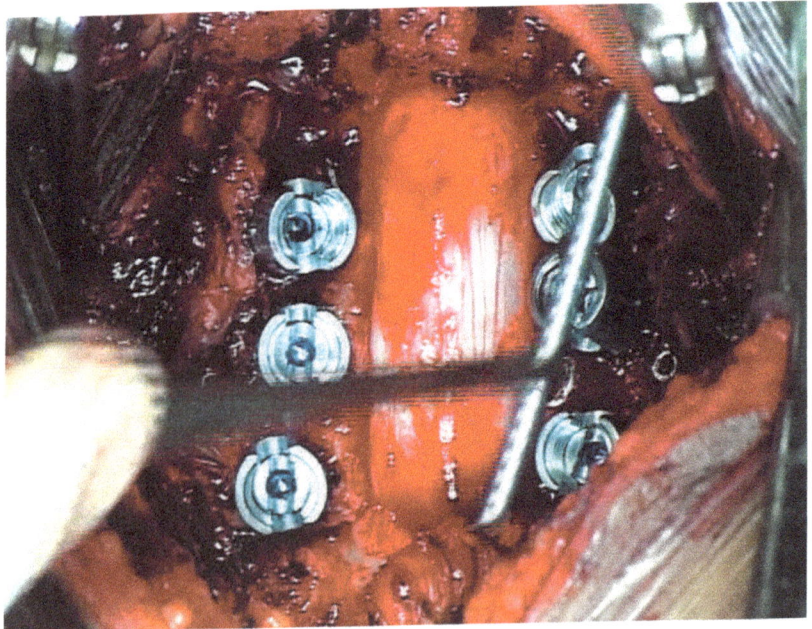

Fig. 8.4 Rod placement checking

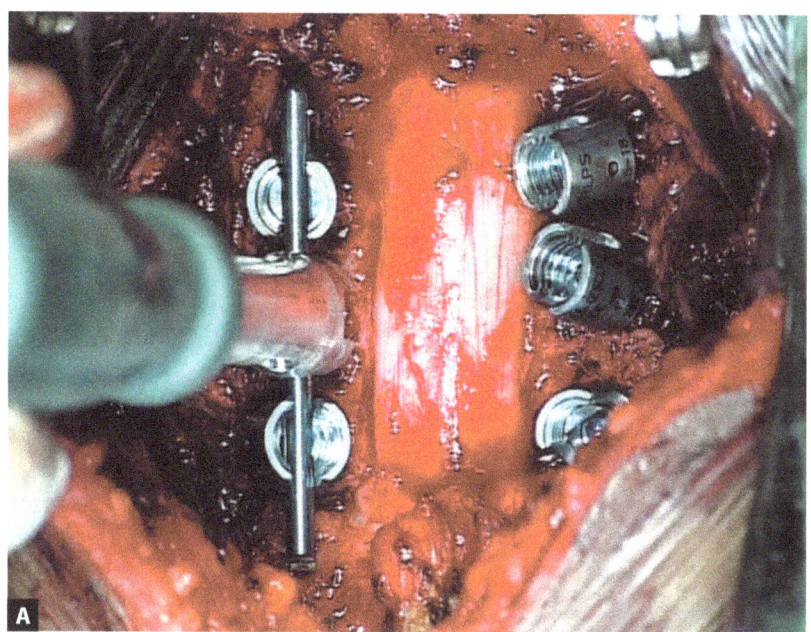
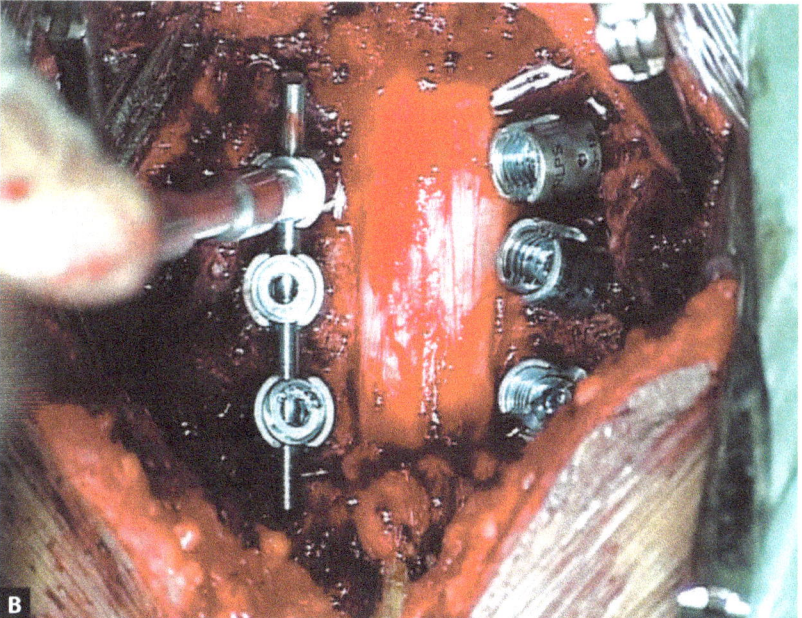

Figs 8.5A and B (A) Securing the innie nut; (B) Securing the innie nut at next site

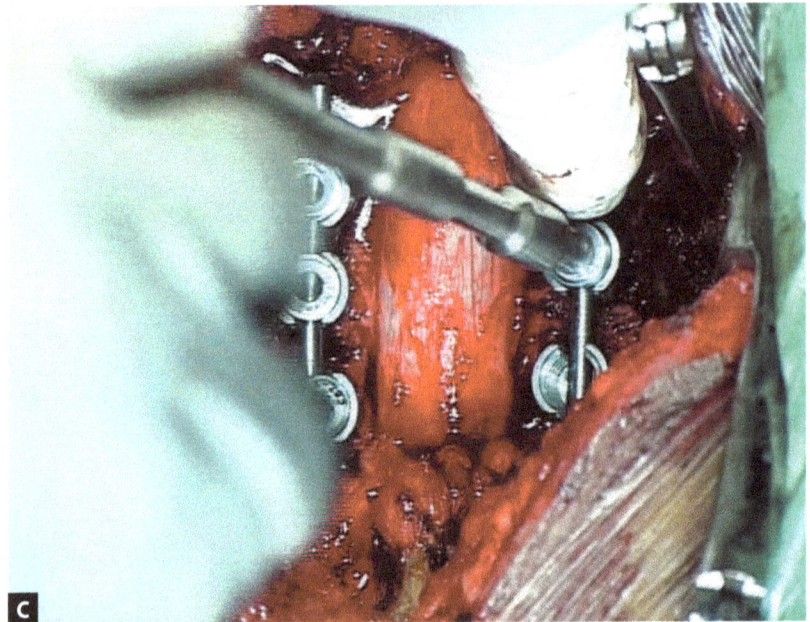
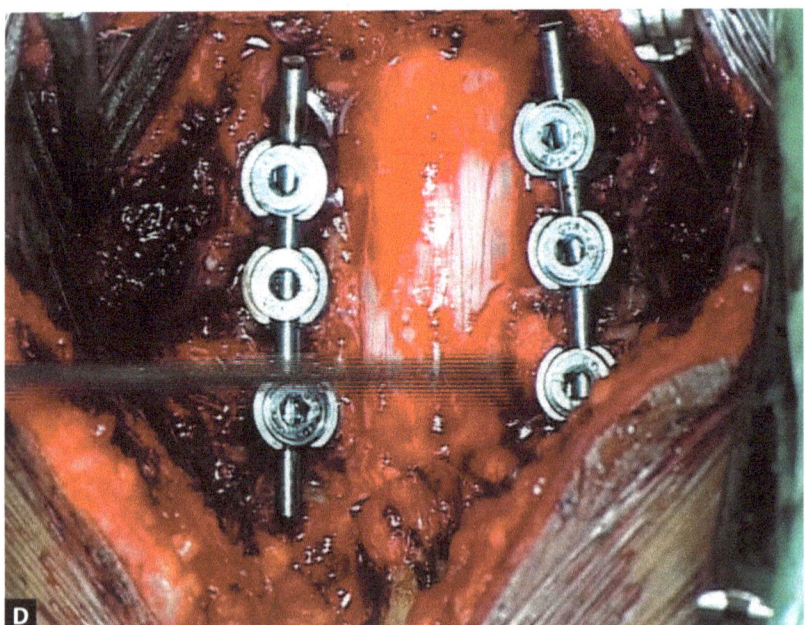

Figs 8.5C and D (C) Securing the innie nut at opposite site;
(D) Firm tightening of the inner check nuts completed

layer is meticulously closed with absorbable suture material and the skin with metal clips **(Fig. 8.7)**.

Chapter 8: Instrumentation

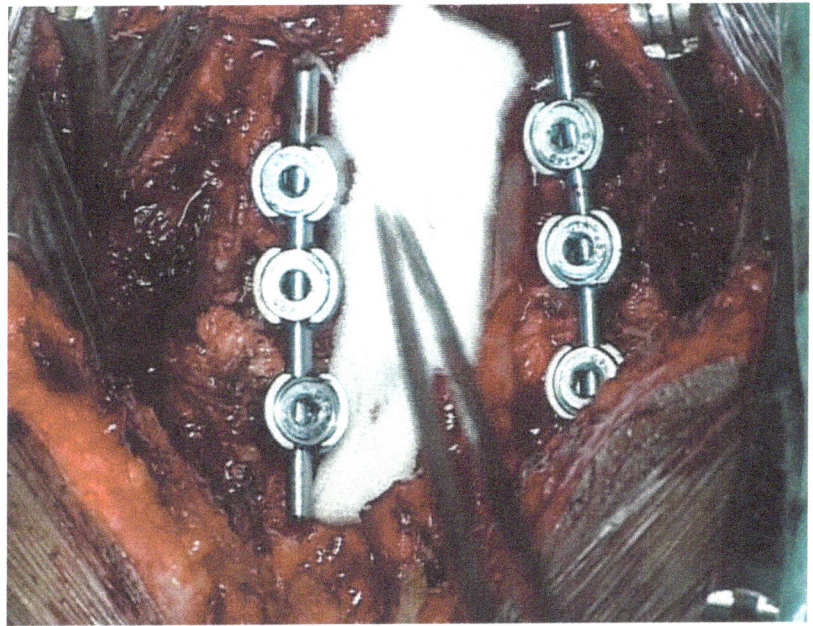

Fig. 8.6 Gelfoam over the dura

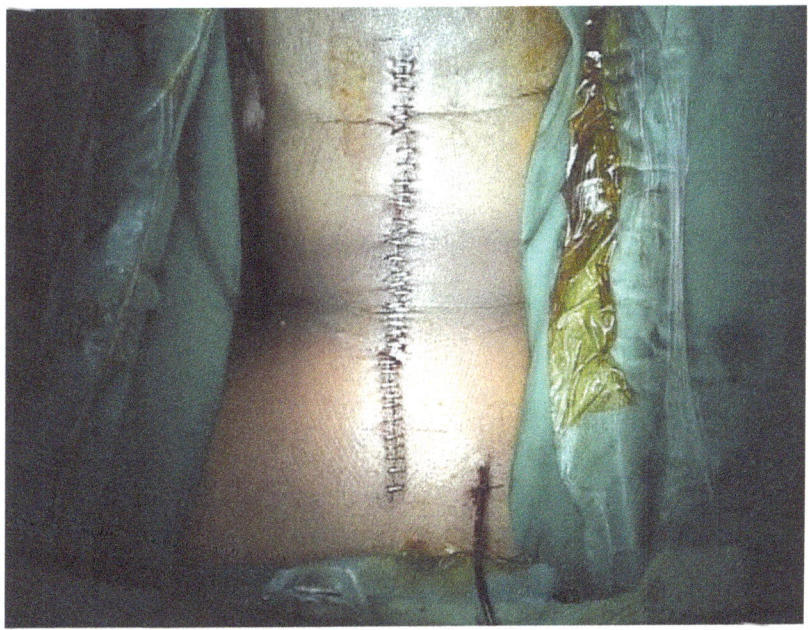

Fig. 8.7 Skin closure with a drain

Chapter 9

Case Reports

CASE 1

Young married woman presented with severe neck pain for one month. She later developed severe pain in the right arm. X-rays of cervical spine showed mild scoliosis and facet erosion at C3 and C4 on the right side **(Fig. 9.1A)**. MRI sagital views demonstrated extradural lesion at C3 and C4 with dural indentation **(Fig. 9.1B)**. Axial views demonstrated significant erosion on right facet joints and granulation tissue extensively **(Fig. 9.1C)**. Posterior approach of cervical region exposed the granulation tissues on right side and normal lateral masses on the left side **(Fig. 9.1D)**. The granulation tissues were removed, the dural layer and nerve root decompressed well. Subsequently, lateral mass screws applied on the left side at C3 and C4 **(Fig. 9.1E)**. Postoperatively patient had excellent pain relief and her follow-up X-rays showed good unilateral fixation **(Fig. 9.1F)**.

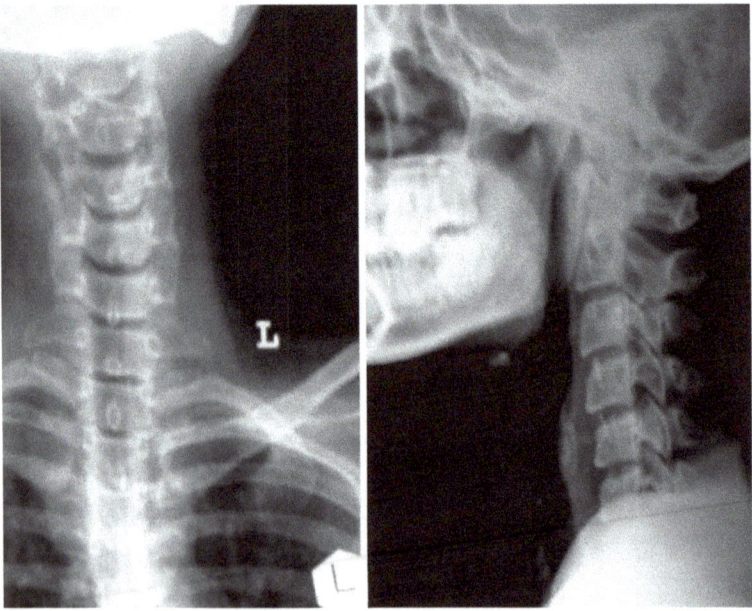

Fig. 9.1A X-ray showing erosion at C3/4 facets and mild scoliosis

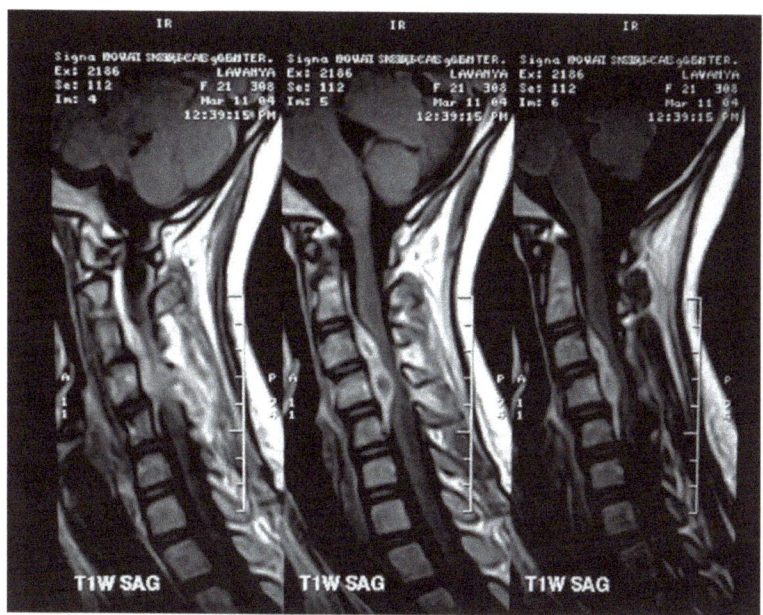

Fig. 9.1B MRI sagittal view showing extradural lesion

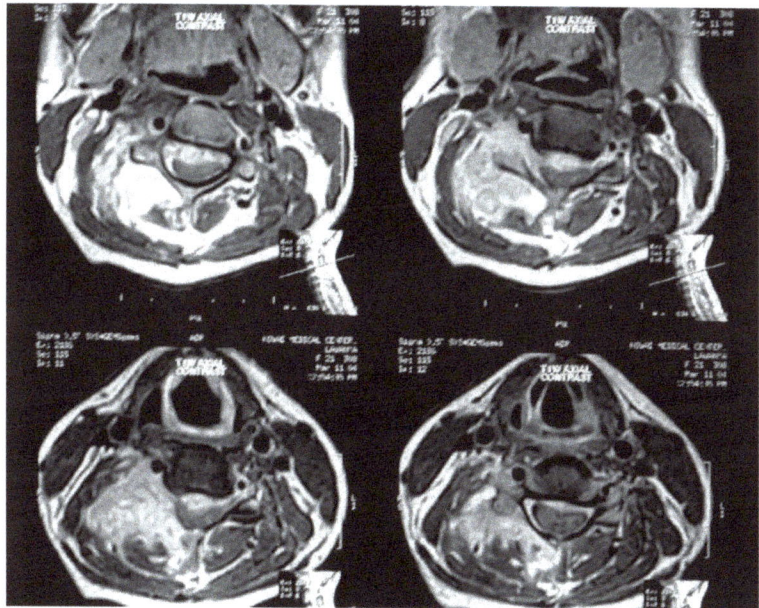

Fig. 9.1C MRI axial cut showing erosion of facets

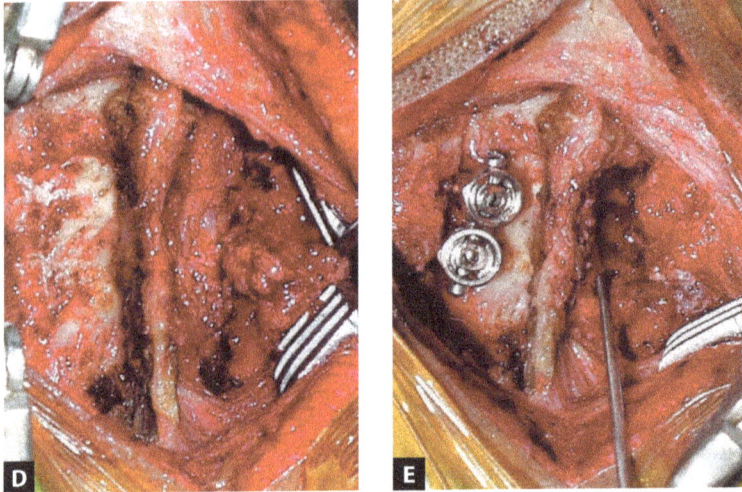

Figs 9.1D and E (D) Preoperative picture showing dense granulation tissue on left side; (E) Preoperative picture showing good neural decompression on right side and lateral mass fixation on left side at C3/4

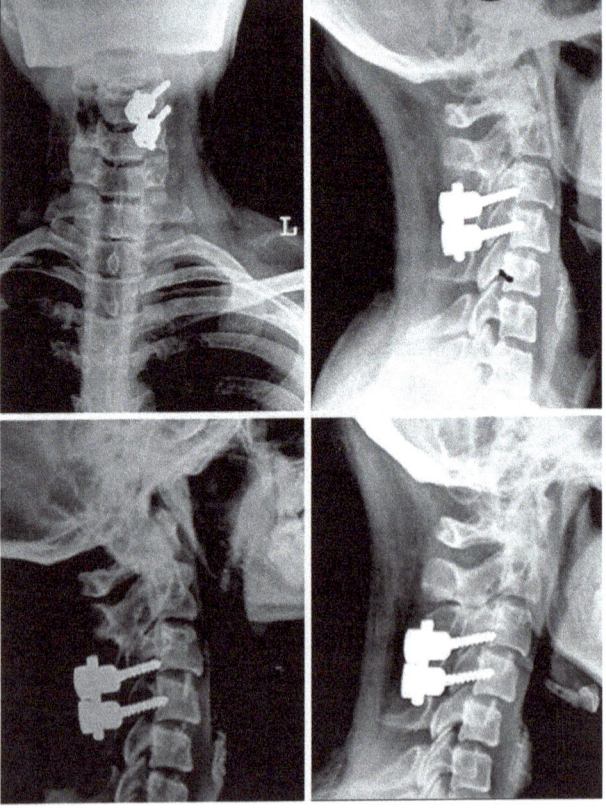

Fig. 9.1F Postoperative follow-up X-ray showing good stabilization

CASE 2

Sixty-year-old obese man with short neck presented to us with progressive difficulty in walking and weakness of hand functions. He had earlier been diagnosed clinically as cervical spondylotic myelopathy earlier and advised to undergo investigations. However, patient had a trivial fall and obtained medical consultation again. This time investigations done showed very severe cervical cord compression at 4 levels from C3 vertebral body to C6/7 disc space level **(Fig. 9.2A)**. He subsequently underwent C3 to C6 spino-laminectomy and C3/4/5/6 lateral mass fixation **(Figs 9.2B to D)**.

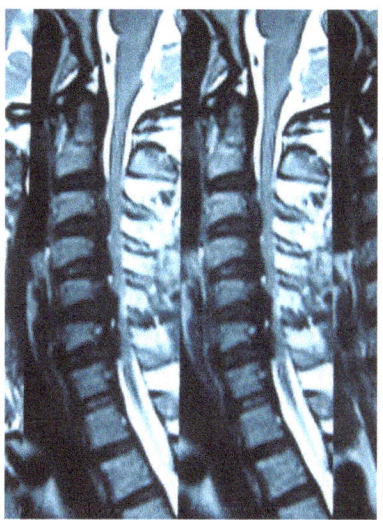

Fig. 9.2A MRI showing significant cord compression from C3 to C6/7

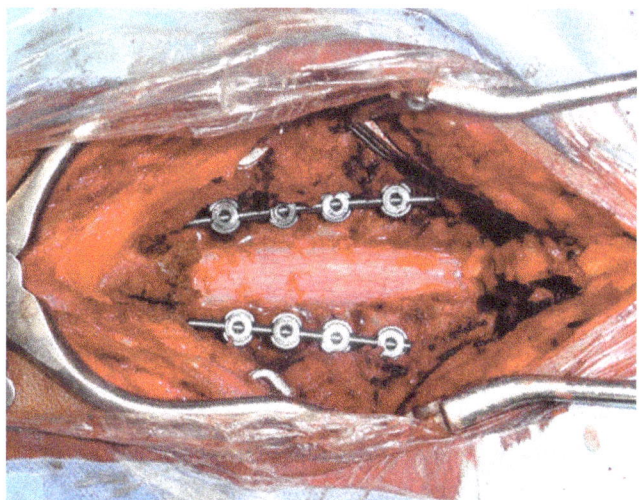

Fig. 9.2B Preoperative picture of spinal laminectomy and lateral mass fixation

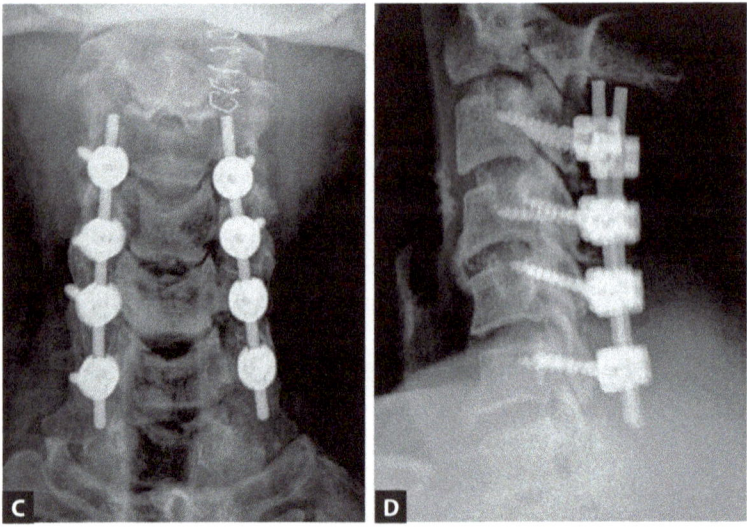

Figs 9.2C and D (C) X-ray anteroposterior view (Note the different lateral angulations); (D) X-ray lateral view (Note the different superior angulations)

CASE 3

Middle aged man sustained severe cervical spine injury in a road traffic accident. He was quadriplegic at the time of admission. Investigations showed C5/6 fracture dislocation with all three segments damaged. There was facet jump with posterior element fractures **(Fig. 9.3A)**. Potentially

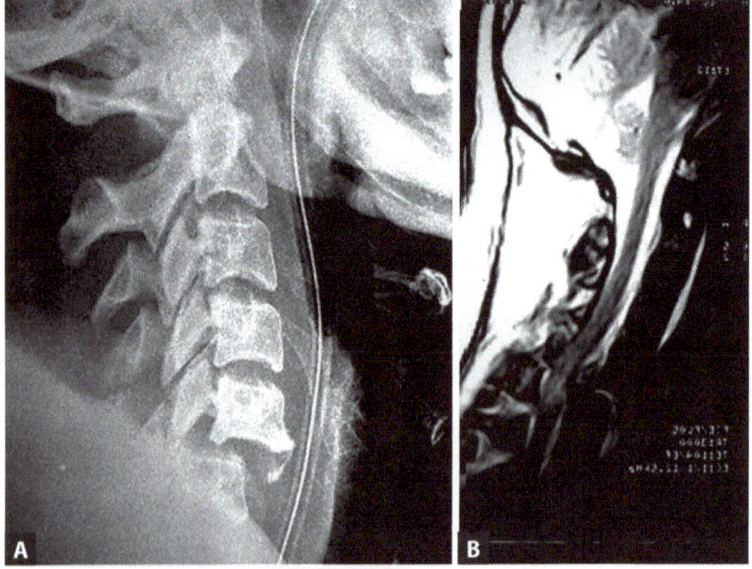

Figs 9.3A and B (A) X-ray showing C5/6 fracture dislocation and all three column damage; (B) MRI showing disc material in the canal

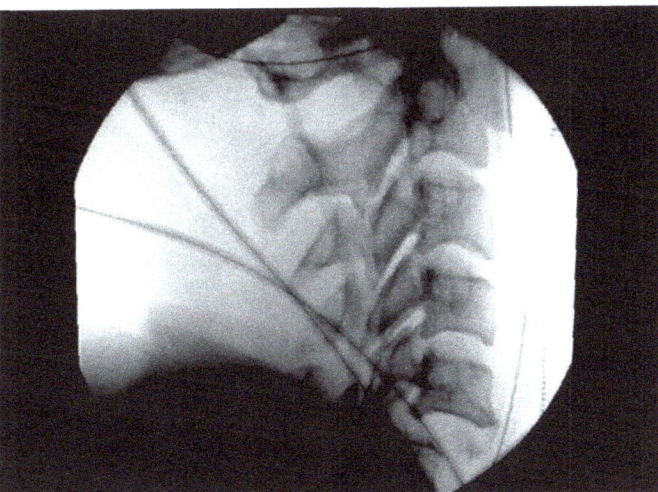

Fig. 9.3C Image intensifier showing irreducible fracture in spite of cervical traction

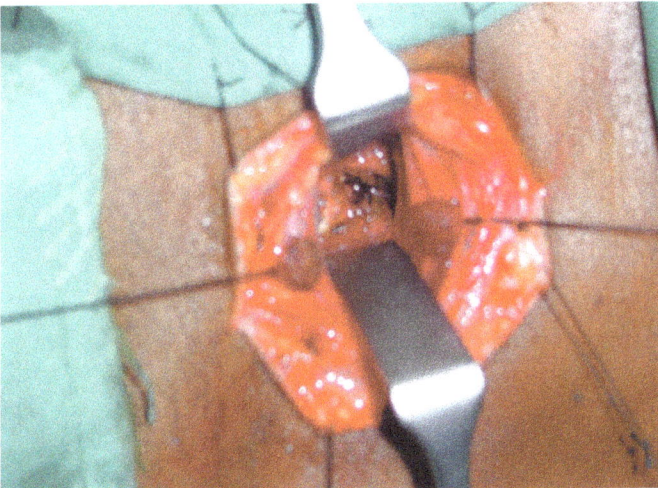

Fig. 9.3D Anterior approach (Stage 1)

unstable with worst neurological condition. Patient had adequate respiration and was conscious. MRI showed cord contusion and compression with the prolapsed disc material in the canal **(Fig. 9.3B)**.

Cervical traction with skull tongs did not reduce the fracture **(Fig. 9.3C)**. Three stage procedure completed the surgical management at the end.

Stage 1: Through an anterolateral approach C5/6 intervertebral disc space exposed and the cartilages removed **(Figs 9.3D and E)**. The dislocation was well appreciated by the step at C5/6 anteriorly. The migrated disc materials were then removed and the dura was seen tented. Intraoperative reduction tried but we could not achieve for obvious reasons. I do not recommend

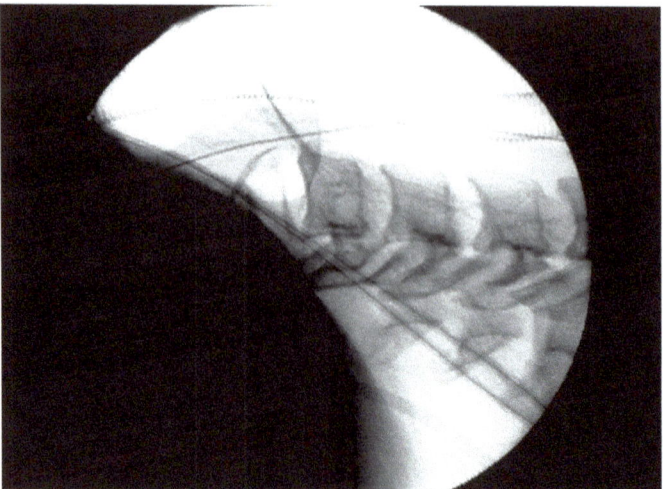

Fig. 9.3E Irreducible dislocation (No force applied)

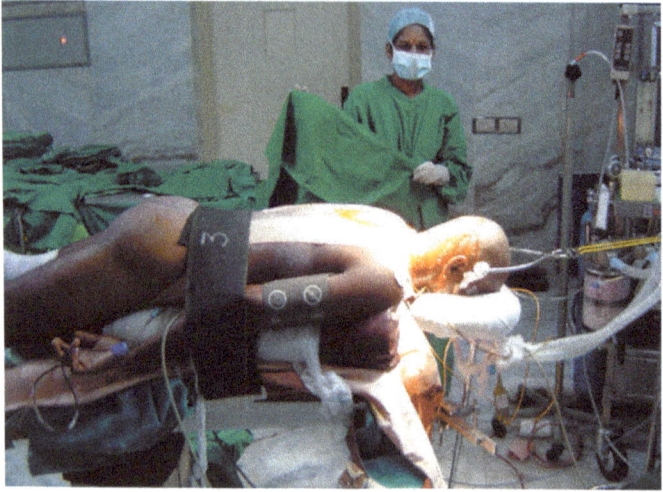

Fig. 9.3F Patient in prone position with skull traction

over distractions to achieve reduction. A reducible dislocation always get reduced with optimum distraction. The anterior wound was closed loose and protected.

Stage 2: Patient was then turned prone and the head placed over the horse shoe rest **(Fig. 9.3F)** and the posterior elements exposed methodically. Superior facets of C6 drilled out and the fracture get reduced by now **(Fig. 9.3G)**. Lateral masses are then drilled and screws placed **(Fig. 9.3H)**.

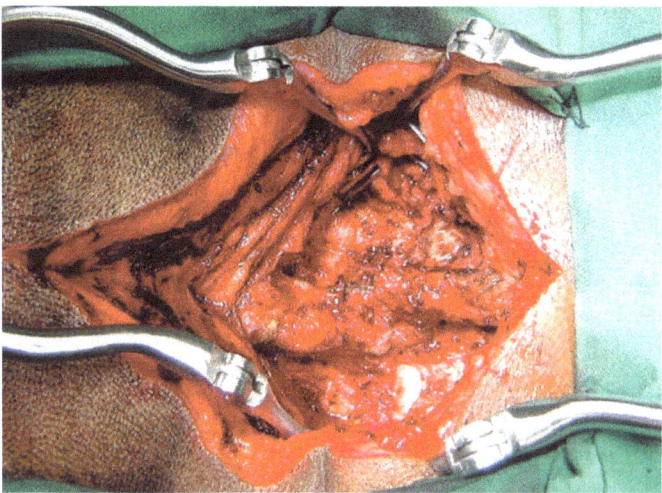

Fig. 9.3G Locked facets

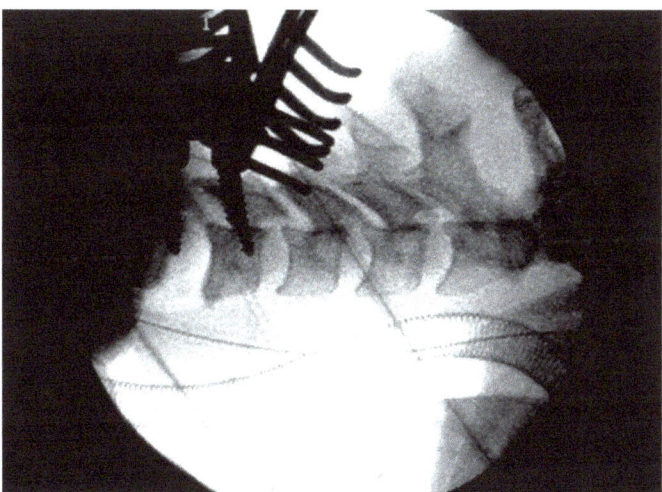

Fig. 9.3H Showing reduction and the screws in place

Reduction and fixation completed with tightening the rods over the screws posterior wound closed in layers **(Fig. 9.3I)**.

Stage 3: Patient is then finally turned to supine again and anterior inter body iliac crest tricortical graft placed and the segment augmented with anterior instrumentation **(Fig. 9.3J)**. This completes the 360°/Global fixation for the three column damage.

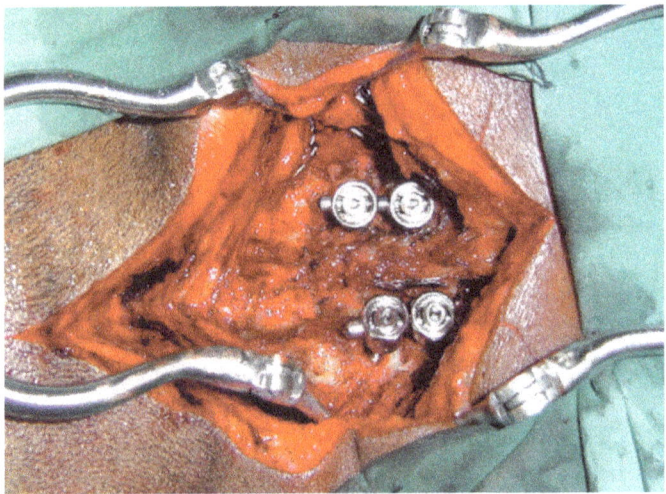

Fig. 9.3I Final fixation with rods

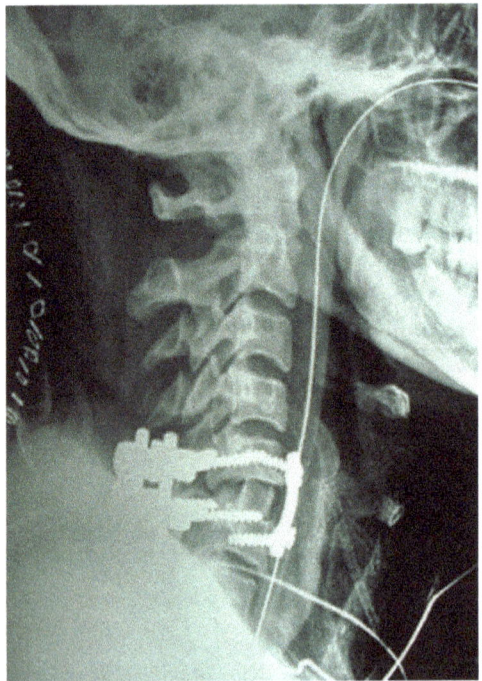

Fig. 9.3J X-ray: Global/360° fixation

CASE 4

Nineteen-year-old girl presented with severe neck pain and progressive torticolis, head tilting to right side. No other symptoms and there were no neurological deficits. She has to hold the neck to be comfortable **(Fig. 9.4A)**. X-rays showed tilt of mandibular angles **(Fig. 9.4B)**. CT showed extensive

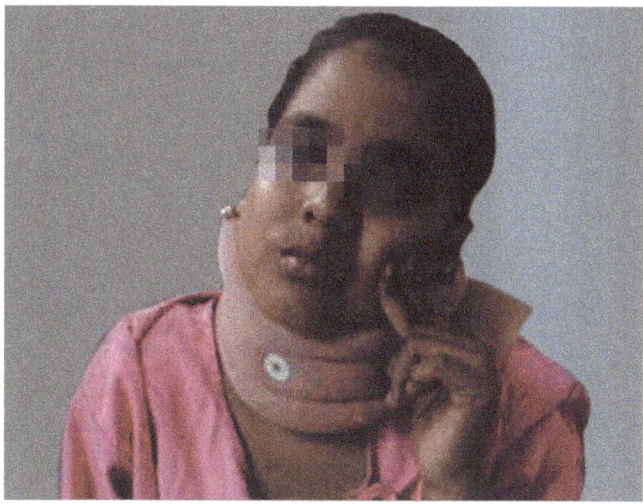

Fig. 9.4A Torticollis and head supported with hands

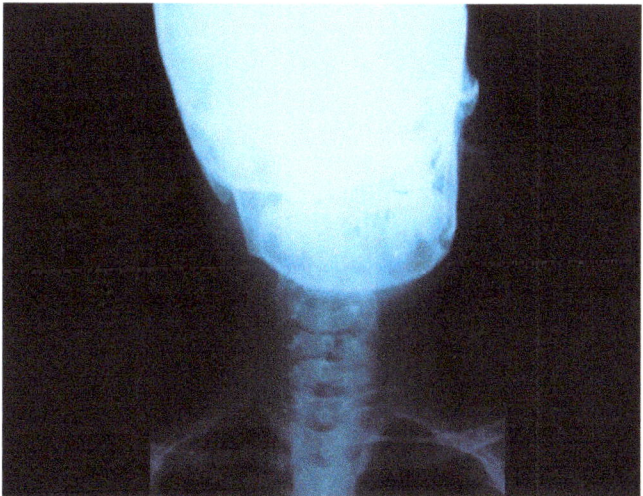

Fig. 9.4B X-ray—anteroposterior view showing Cock Hen neck appearance

bony erosion and destruction of right lateral mass of C1 with collapse of the Occipito atlanto axial component on right side resulting subluxation of the C1/2 joint on the left side with a tilt and rotation **(Fig. 9.4C)**. No doubt that patient needed external support to prevent excruciating pain. MRI showed the same findings along with granulation tissues that encroach the canal though the cord was not compressed **(Fig. 9.4D)**. Transverse ligament was not seen well.

She underwent Occipito extended cervical fixation and grafting **(Figs 9.4E and F)**. Lateral mass screws were placed in C3 and C4 and

54 Section 2: Surgical Techniques

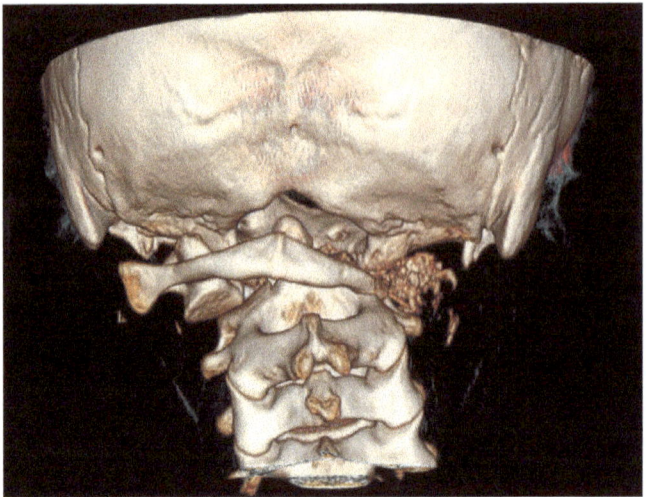

Fig. 9.4C CT 3D reconstruction image showing erosion of lateral mass of C1 on left side

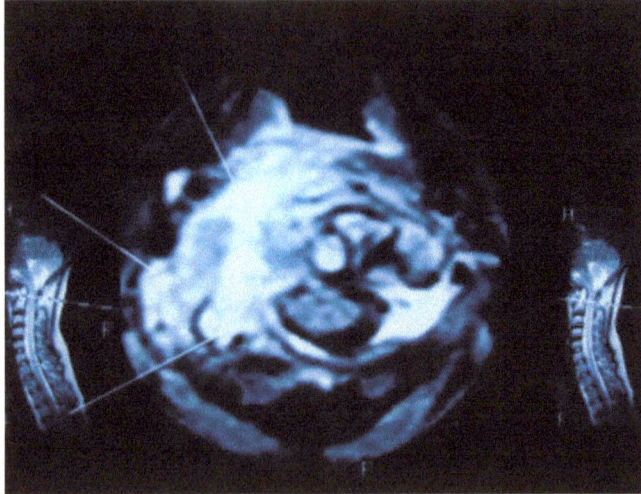

Fig. 9.4D MRI showing the granulation tissues in the canal

predesigned rods then connected and fixed to occipital bone with screws **(Fig. 9.4G)**. The provision for instrumentation at C1 and C2 were not possible. Torticolis got corrected and completely relieved the patient of pain in the first postoperative day itself. Antituberculosis drugs were given for programmed period.

Chapter 9: Case Reports 55

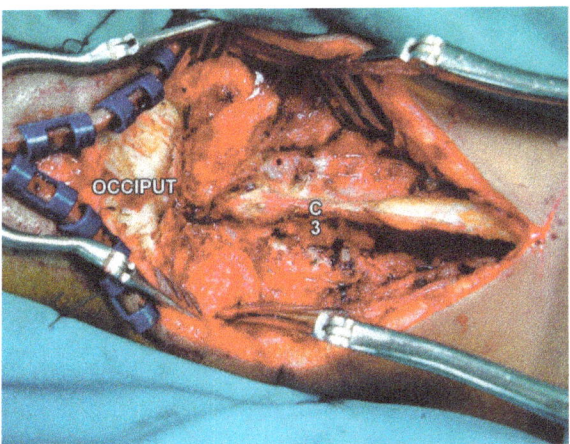

Fig. 9.4E Exposure of occiput and C3/4 lateral masses

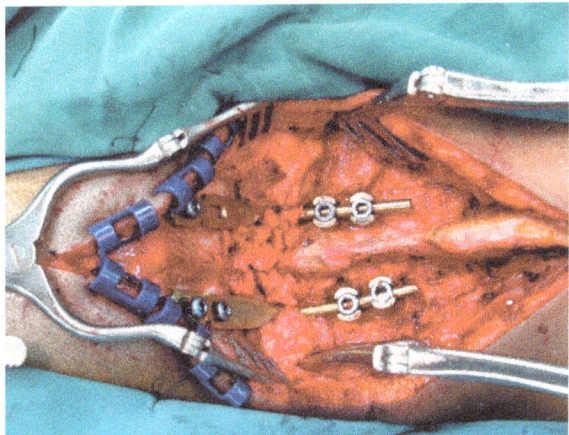

Fig. 9.4F Occiput extended cervical fixation with bone grafting over C1/2 posteriorly

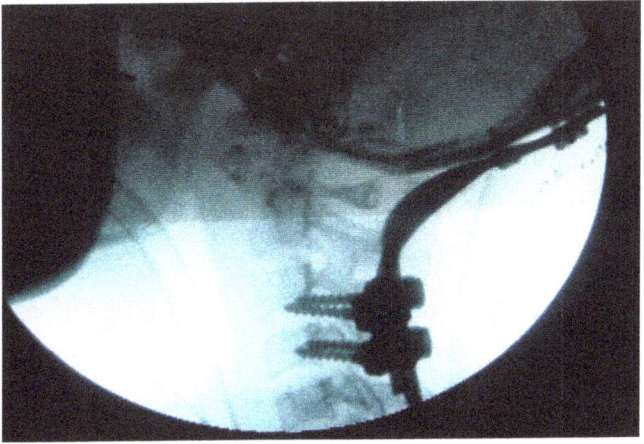

Fig. 9.4G X-ray lateral view showing the instrumentation

56 Section 2: Surgical Techniques

CASE 5

This is a similar case as the previous one. A middle aged man who had severe neck pain and needed to support his neck all the time **(Fig. 9.5A)**. There was a significant torticolis X-ray showed classical picture **(Fig. 9.5B)**. CT showed extensive erosion of C1 lateral mass on the left side **(Figs 9.5C to E)** and MRI showed signal changes indicative of granulation tissue **(Fig. 9.5F)**. In this case it was less severe than the previous patient. However, the pain and discomfort was significant for this office going gentleman.

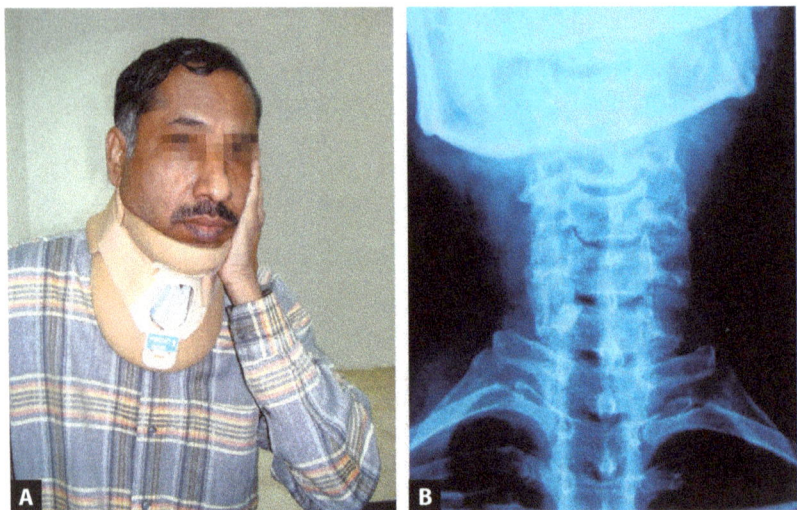

Figs 9.5A and B (A) Torticollis and hand holding the head; (B) X-ray—anteroposterior view showing Cock Hen neck appearance

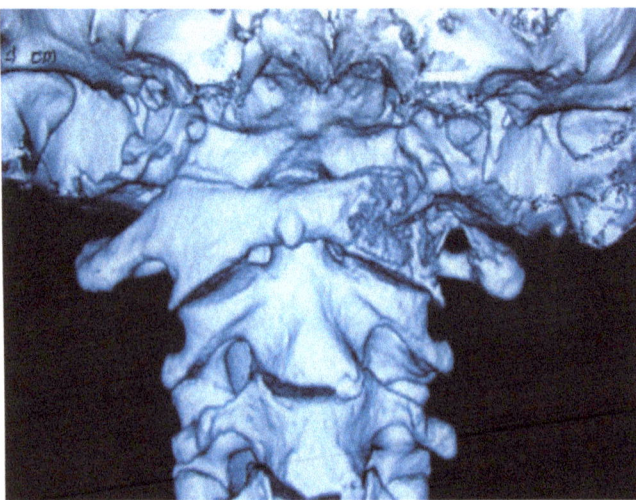

Fig. 9.5C CT 3D reconstruction showing erosion of C1 lateral mass

Chapter 9: Case Reports 57

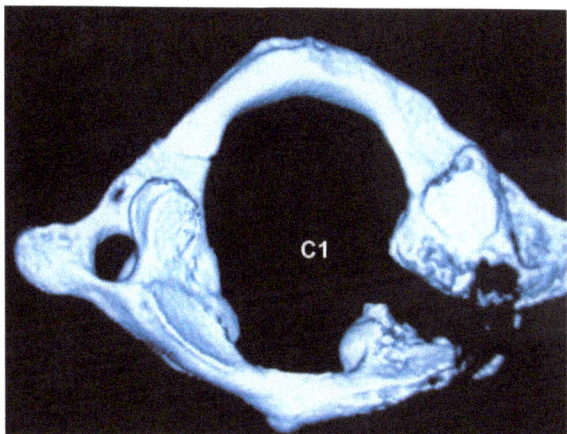

Fig. 9.5D CT axial views showing the erosion anterior arch

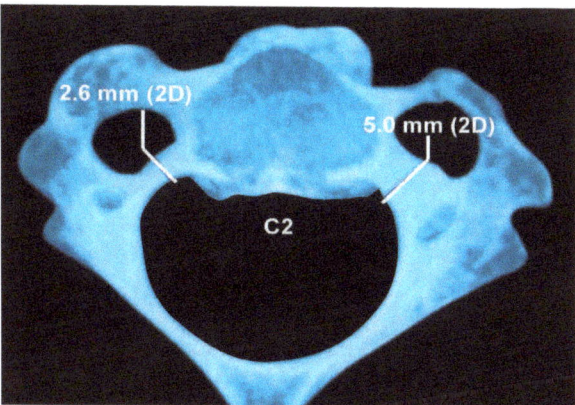

Fig. 9.5E CT axial cut C2 showing narrow pedicles

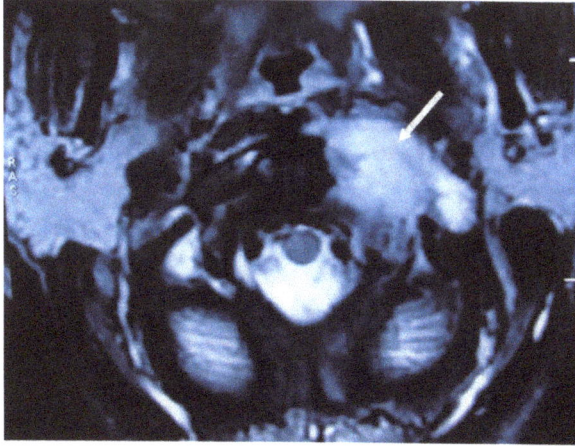

Fig. 9.5F MRI showing granulation tissue, canal spared

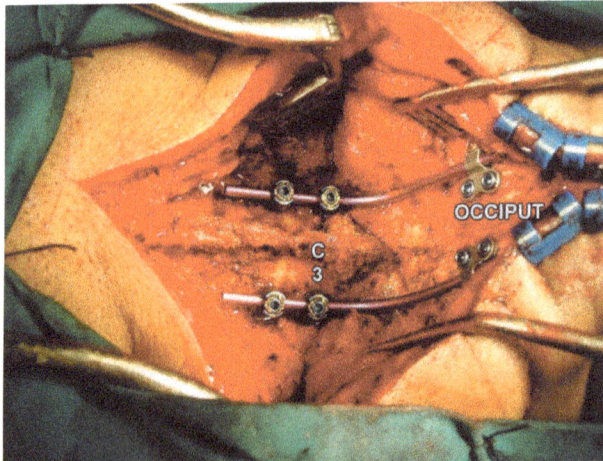

Fig. 9.5G Occiput extended C3/4 lateral mass fixation

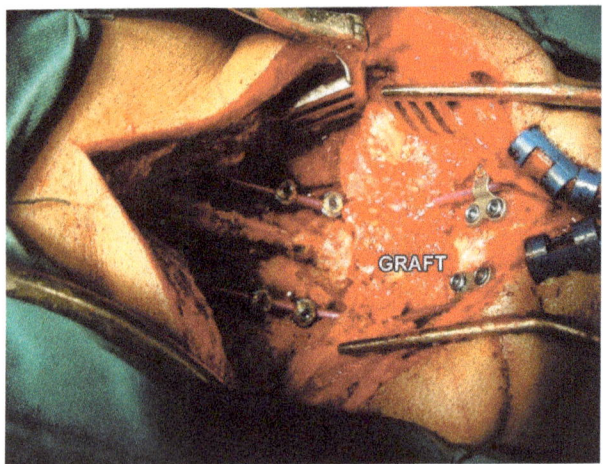

Fig. 9.5H CI/2 posterior grafting

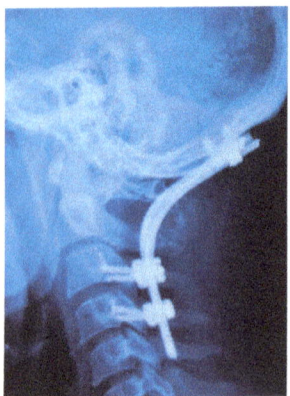

Fig. 9.5I X-ray—lateral view showing the instrumentation

He underwent occipito extended cervical fusion resulting in good recovery from pain **(Figs 9.5G to I)**.

CASE 6

A case of multilevel ossification of the posterior longitudinal ligament (OPLL) operated with lateral mass fixation along with miniplate expansion laminoplasty following a failed anterior approach **(Figs 9.6A and B)**.

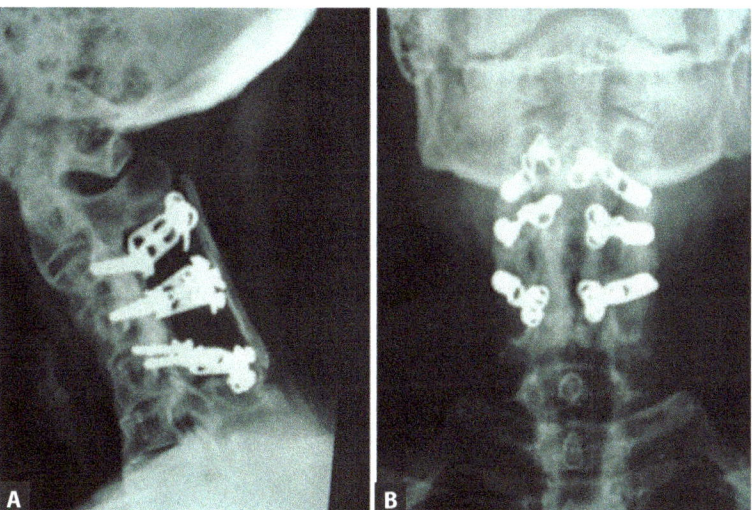

Figs 9.6A and B (A) X-ray—lateral view postoperative-lateral mass screws and miniplates with supraspinous iliac graft; (B) X-ray anteroposterior view showing the miniplates in expansion laminoplasty

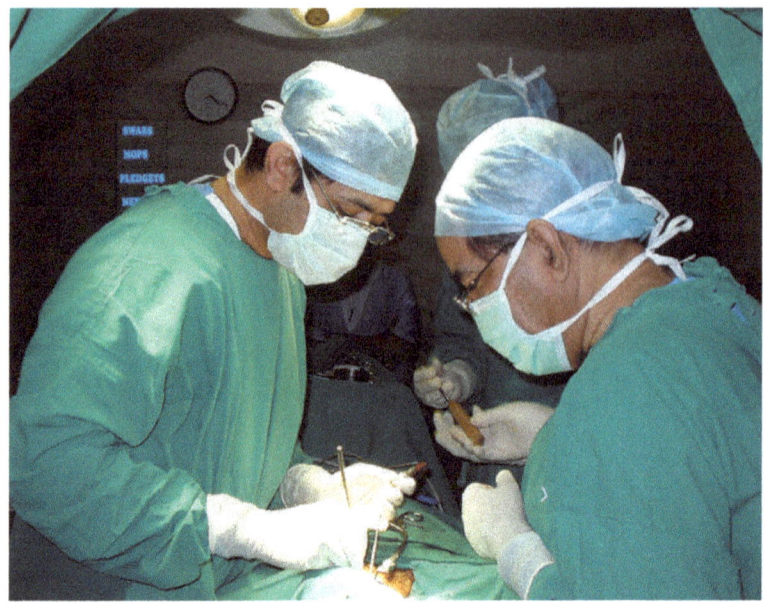

My heart says 'I am grateful to my Mentor and Guru for encouraging me to become a teacher for younger generations to come. One should start learning the alphabets before writing a poem. Thank you Professor PS Ramani'

Index

Page numbers followed by *f* refer to figure and *t* refer to table

A

Angulation of superior facet 4*f*
Articular facet
    inferior 4*f*
    superior 4*f*
Articular pillar 3, 4*f*

B

Bladder catheter compressor 20*f*

C

C1 lateral mass 56*f*
C1 on left side 54*f*
C1/2 posterior grafting 58*f*
C3/4 lateral mass fixation 58*f*
C5/6 fracture dislocation 48*f*
Cervical fixation with bone grafting over
    C1/2 posteriorly 55*f*
Cervical nerve roots 9, 9*f*
Cervical spine, alignment of 24*f*
Cock hen neck 53*f*, 56*f*
Cord compression from C3 to C6/7 47*f*
Cranial nerve roots 6
CT 3D reconstruction 54*f*
CT axial cut C2 narrow pedicles 57*f*

D

Dense granulation tissue on left side 46*f*
Disc material in canal 48*f*
Drill hole site 33*f*, 34*f*
Drilling 32
    outer cortex diamond burr 32*f*

E

Endotracheal general anesthesia 19
Endotracheal tube 22*t*
Erosion anterior arch 57*f*
Erosion at C3/4 facets and mild
    scoliosis 44*f*
Expansion laminoplasty 59*f*
Extradural lesion 45*f*

F

Facet
    erosion of 45*f*
    locked 51
Facet joint
    graft bed preparation of 35*f*
    grafting 39*f*
    inspection 27*f*
        opposite site 28*f*
Fixation with bicortical screws 15*f*
Flexometallic endotracheal tube 19*f*
Foramen transversarium 3, 12

G

Global/360° fixation 52*f*

H

Hillock 5*f*
    and foramen transversarium 11*f*

I

Innie nut at opposite site 42*f*
Intensifier on floor 24

Intrafacet line 8
Irreducible dislocation 50*f*

J

Joint 4*f*

L

Lateral border marked 28*f*
Lateral facet line 8
Lateral margin of lamina 5*f*
Ligaments and facet joints 25

M

Magerl entry point 14*f*
Magerl technique 13
Mayfield three-pin head clamp 20*f*
Medial facet line 8
Midline nuchal fascia cut with scissors 25*f*
Midline skin mark 23*f*
Miniplates with supraspinous iliac graft 59*f*
Monopolar cautery 30*f*, 31*f*

N

Neck skin folding 22*f*
Nerve drawn with pen 9*f*
Neurovascular structures 15*f*
   anterior to lateral mass 6*f*
   in relation to lateral mass 9

O

Occiput and C3/4 lateral masses 55*f*

P

Paraspinal muscles 23, 25, 26*f*, 38

R

Rod placement checking 40*f*
Rods, final fixation with 52*f*
Rostrocaudal line 8

S

Saline irrigation while drilling 35*f*
Screw trajectories and critical points 13
Skin closure with drain 43*f*
Skull traction 50*f*
Spinal laminectomy and lateral mass
   fixation 47*f*
Standard screw trajectories 13
Subaxial cervical spine 4*f*
Subcutaneous tissue 25
Superior facet joint 29*f*
Surgical anatomy of lateral mass 3

T

Tissues in canal 54*f*
Torticollis
   and hand holding head 56*f*
   and head supported with hands 53*f*

V

Vertebral artery position 11*f*

www.ingramcontent.com/pod-product-compliance
Lightning Source LLC
Chambersburg PA
CBHW040518220526
45473CB00012B/2900